THE
MEMORY
BIBLE

THE
MEMORY
BIBLE

Secrets of a Super Memory
and Optimal Brain Health

EARL L. MINDELL,
R.PH., M.H., PH.D.

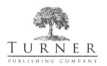

TURNER
PUBLISHING COMPANY

Turner Publishing Company
424 Church Street • Suite 2240 • Nashville, Tennessee 37219
445 Park Avenue • 9th Floor • New York, New York 10022
www.turnerpublishing.com

Library of Congress Cataloging-in-Publication Data

Mindell, Earl.
    Dr. Earl Mindell's memory bible : secrets of a super memory and optimal brain health / Earl L. Mindell, R.Ph., M.H., Ph.D.
      pages cm
    Includes bibliographical references and index.
    ISBN 978-1-59120-398-8
1. Memory—Nutritional aspects. 2. Memory disorders—Prevention. 3. Intellect—Nutritional aspects. 4. Brain—Care and hygiene. 5. Dietary supplements. 6. Cognition in old age. 7. Memory in old age. I. Title.
    QP406.M56   2015
    612.8'23312—dc23

                            2014049030

Editor: Carol Killman Rosenberg
Typesetting and cover design: Gary A. Rosenberg

Printed in the United States of America

10 9 8 7 6 5 4 3 2 1

Contents

Why You Need a Memory Supplement

Today, 4.5 million Americans and 35 million people worldwide are impacted by age-related memory and cognition problems. By 2050, the number worldwide is expected to climb beyond 115 million. Fifteen new cases of dementia are diagnosed every minute.

Human life expectancy has increased by about eight years in only five decades. Dementia is becoming a serious problem because we are living longer life spans than ever before, and the diseases that once did us in before we experienced loss of memory and decreased thinking ability are no longer life-threatening. More people survive well into their eighties and beyond than ever before. They want to live full, involved, independent lives, which requires good cognitive function.

Dementia is chronic and progressive. Its future increase here in the United States and in other countries—especially developing countries—stands to wreak havoc on the ability of younger generations to manage its economic and caregiver impact.

The good news is that there is a lot we can do to forestall the brain changes that lead to cognitive decline. We know a great deal about the factors that most strongly influence brain aging. And you'll be surprised to learn how many very commonly prescribed medications—drugs being taken by the majority of those over seventy years old in some parts of the world—may be contributing to the epidemic of premature cognitive decline. Exercise is particularly potent here—only an hour a week appears to cut the risk of Alzheimer's disease in half.

Before we begin looking at solutions, let's take a look at the most common memory and cognition issues people tend to face as they age.

DEMENTIA

This is a catchall term describing any form of cognitive decline. The most common cause of age-related dementia is Alzheimer's disease, but it can also be triggered by one or more small strokes, which can cause cumulative damage that has symptoms like those of Alzheimer's. The only way to know for sure whether dementia is specifically of the Alzheimer's variety or is due to other causes is to actually look at an individual's brain tissue postmortem, as Dr. Alzheimer did with his first patient (see below).

ALZHEIMER'S DISEASE (AD)

In 1906, Bavarian physician Alois Alzheimer identified the first defined case of what he called "presenile dementia." The patient gradually lost her ability to form and retain short-term memories, and developed other symptoms too, including agitation. After her death, Dr. Alzheimer dissected her brain and found deposits of a substance called beta-amyloid, along with *neurofibrillary tangles,* or clumps of damaged neurons, in a part of the brain called the hippocampus. This was the first documented case of the disease that now is responsible for 60 to 80 percent of dementia cases.

Most people who develop AD are sixty-five or older, but up to 5 percent of people who have the disease fall into the category of "early onset"—they begin to have symptoms in their forties or fifties.

Alzheimer's disease is a progressive disease that worsens over time. On average, a person can expect to live between four and twenty years following the point at which his or her symptoms become obvious. Life expectancy for someone with AD also depends on the person's overall health and the presence or absence of other health conditions. Alzheimer's disease is the sixth leading cause of death in the United States.

Modern medicine does not have a cure for AD. Medical treatments do exist, and they vary in effectiveness. Research into both alternative and mainstream therapies is ongoing, as are investigations designed to help create preventive programs or to slow down the progression of the disease once it is diagnosed. Sometimes, the best that can be done is to improve quality of life for the person with AD and to help keep caregivers' responsibilities manageable.

The risk of AD is substantially increased by several of the same activities and factors we know to increase risk of heart disease and cancer:

- Physical inactivity increases risk of AD by 82 percent.

- Depression increases risk 65 percent.

- Hypertension (high blood pressure) in midlife increases risk by 61 percent.

- Obesity in midlife increases risk by 60 percent.

- Smoking increases risk by 59 percent.

- Diabetes increases risk by 46 percent.

The damage that ultimately leads to AD symptoms begins to develop a decade or more before those symptoms appear. Damage seen in AD involves inflammation, oxidative stress, loss of mitochondrial resources, and insulin resistance in brain cells (also called neurons). Together, these factors contribute to creating atrophy and damage in nerve cells crucial for learning and short-term memory.

I'll go into more detail about all these factors later in this book. The important basics, for now, are that all of these factors are strongly influenced by diet and lifestyle. It is theorized that the buildup of amyloid, a protein substance, in the brain—the thing believed to gum up the works in AD—is actually a part of an immune response gone awry. Modern unhealthy diets depleted of crucial nutrients "trick" the body into sending overblown immune defenses to tissues where they end up doing more harm than good.

Diets high in sugars, other refined carbohydrates, and unhealthy fats, and low in whole plant foods push blood sugar balance in an unhealthy direction, setting the stage for type 2 diabetes (which is expected to be diagnosed in nearly half of adults in the United States in their lifetimes). Type 2 diabetes and its precursor, insulin resistance, lead to chronically high blood sugars and insulin levels. This, in turn, worsens every physiologic circumstance that contributes to AD. People with diabetes who control their blood sugar, eat a really healthy diet, and exercise can do a lot to slow cognitive decline and delay a potential AD diagnosis.

SENIOR MOMENTS:
AN INEVITABLE PART OF AGING?

You forget the name of a lifelong friend. You miss an appointment. You can't remember your ATM PIN number. You go upstairs to get something, then can't remember what you had planned to get. You misplace your car keys. "Senior moment!" you say. But how do these moments really feel?

Depending on how much your mental acuity means to you, you might experience a chuckle of recognition, a shock of real fear, or some combination of the two. If you aren't sure whether this is a harbinger of more serious memory and cognition problems, your feelings might be more along the lines of mortal terror.

Let me allay any fears you might have that "senior moments" are linked to AD or other kinds of dementia. Scientists have traced these lapses in memory or thinking back to a decline in a specific protein in the brain called RbAp48. Levels of this protein in the hippocampus, the same part of the brain impacted by AD, decline as we age. Minor senior moments that don't interfere significantly in your day-to-day life are not likely to suggest dementia setting in.

Some of the more exciting aspects of this research suggest that restoring RbAp48 in the hippocampus could help restore cognitive function lost with the passage of time.

If you do have concerns about mental fogginess or forgetfulness indicating a more serious problem, enlist friends and loved ones to give you feedback about how forgetful you seem to them over time. Do they see a worsening of the problem? If so, something called *mild cognitive impairment* (MCI)—a middle ground between AD and senior moments—may be setting in. It's sensible to get evaluated by a physician if you suspect you may have MCI.

Simple steps like getting enough sleep, engaging in healthy coping strategies in response to stress, eating well, using targeted nutritional supplementation, and keeping your brain active and engaged will help prevent senior moments from getting the best of you. So does more mindfulness—paying more intense attention to the sensory details of what is going on around you. Don't try to multitask. Allow new memories to form more vividly as you move through your life, and engage in practices like mental rehearsal or replay of things you want to make sure you remember.

I'd also recommend going easy on yourself in terms of your expectations that you should be able to stay on top of everything this busy world throws your way. In this digital age, our day-to-day responsibilities and the number of things we're expected to track and remember has ballooned to a point where even a sharp thirty-year-old has to struggle to manage it all.

THE BRAIN INITIATIVE
(Brain Research Through Advancing Innovative Neurotechnologies)

This book comes to you during quite an exciting time in the study of the human brain. The federal government has committed $100 billion in funding toward scientific endeavors aimed at gaining a better understanding of this miraculous and mysterious three-pound chunk of nervous system tissue.

The BRAIN Initiative is analogous to the Human Genome Project, which began in the 1980s and culminated in the early 2000s with publication of the sequencing of 90 percent of the 3 billion base pairs contained in the human genome. That project revealed an astonishing amount of information that has aided medical science in understanding, preventing, and treating human diseases, and we have every reason to expect that this concerted effort to understand the workings of the human brain will have a similar impact.

The BRAIN Initiative will enroll the best and brightest research minds across disciplines, bringing them together in collaborations that will enrich our understanding of the brain's function and the ways in which damage occurs. It will help us broaden and deepen our understanding of the biological foundations of mental processes, which will help us understand and treat mood disorders, autism spectrum disorders, and other common issues. We'll better understand how we think, feel, perceive, and remember, and we'll be able to translate that understanding into more effective prevention and treatment of brain issues across the whole life span.

The sooner we begin to mindfully impact as many of these factors as possible through targeted nutrition and lifestyle changes (including replacing brain-draining prescription drugs with nutritional supplements and dietary choices that make them no longer necessary), the longer we're likely to hang on to our mental sharpness and our precious memories, and to *not* create unnecessary burdens for our children and grandchildren.

Even now, so many adults who are raising their own kids have become members of the so-called "sandwich generation," acting simultaneously as caregivers for their offspring and for their aging parents whose cognitive decline makes living on their own too risky a proposition. No one should have to be in the middle of *that* sandwich. It's a terribly stressful place to be, and it can certainly increase stress and compromise health for people who are in a life stage where good health should be a given.

I, for one, hope to live at least a century in good health and with my mental faculties intact! So far, I'm staying at the top of my game, and in these pages I'll share with you a comprehensive plan for doing the same for yourself. My advice is drawn from my lifelong work as a pharmacist, an herbal expert, and an author of dozens of books, booklets, and articles about nutritional supplements and alternatives to prescription drugs.

I'm happy to be your guide on this journey. Let's begin.

For more information, log onto www.nowfoods.com/
RememBrain-60veg-capsules.htm

1

Drugs That Can Cause Memory Loss and Reduce Cognitive Function

'm a big fan of modern medicine when it's needed. Antibiotics, vaccines, and other modern pharmaceuticals have extended life spans, reduced suffering, and improved quality of life for countless people over the past century. And as a pharmacist and expert on alternatives to prescription drugs, I know well that modern medicine, like just about anything that's good, is best in moderation.

Since I began writing, speaking, and learning in the 1970s, the fundamental truth of it all hasn't changed: When we overuse or become unnecessarily dependent on drugs—or when we confuse the tamping-down of symptoms with medications with the actual rebalancing and self-care that really improve and sustain health—we're playing a losing game. Today, prescription drugs are such a big part of most people's lives that we tend to think they help without harming. Our trust in these products is so great that 88 percent of people aged sixty and over take at least one prescription drug on a regular basis. Over a third take *five or more*. Almost 45 percent of people over sixty now take prescription medicines that lower cholesterol—double the rate of use in 1999.

Drugs are designed to target very specific aspects of physiologic function. And when we go into a complex set of systems like those that make up the human body and change a single aspect, we disrupt the other parts of that system. That's why every drug has side effects. Some of these side effects are minor; others are potentially life threatening. And the side effects of some drugs include disruption of memory and cognition.

If you are on these medications, chances are good that the doctor who prescribes them or the pharmacist who dispenses them will give you a heads-up about the possibility of these side effects. So it's especially important for you, as an educated consumer, to know that these medicines could be impacting your ability to think and remember. It's also important for you to know that there are natural alternatives to many of these pharmaceuticals—alternatives your doctor is unlikely to offer to you, because their mind-set tends to be that most people won't do what is necessary to maintain or restore their health. Sadly, this is true of many folks. But since you're reading this book to learn about natural ways to support cognitive function, I'm guessing that you are the exception to that rule.

DRUGS THAT CAN INTERFERE WITH OR CAUSE LOSS OF MEMORY: AN OVERVIEW

antidepressants	muscle relaxants
antihistamines	pain medications given after surgery
benzodiazepines (anti-anxiety medications)	sleeping pills
cholesterol-lowering drugs (statins)	tranquilizers

All of the drugs described in this chapter can create or worsen memory loss or interfere with brain function. Let's look at what they are, what they're prescribed for, and how you might be able to reduce or eliminate your need for them through healthier lifestyle choices and nutritional supplementation.

ANTI-ANXIETY DRUGS (BENZODIAZEPINES)

"Benzos" are prescribed to treat anxiety disorders, agitation, and muscle spasms. They are also used to prevent seizures and help relieve insomnia. They work by reducing the activity of certain areas of the brain—including those parts of the brain that transfer memories from short-term to long-term storage. When benzodiazepines are added to the cocktail of drugs administered during anesthesia, they help erase any unpleasant memories a patient might have as a result of the procedure.

As is the case with most psychiatric drugs, benzodiazepine prescriptions are on the rise. They are often combined with opioid analgesics (strong painkillers that also have a tranquilizing effect) and are increasingly prescribed in primary-care practices. In a Centers for Disease Control (CDC) study involving 3.1 billion primary-care visits between 2002 and 2009, 12.6 percent involved prescriptions for benzodiazepines or opioids (a related drug class). During that time period, prescriptions of benzodiazepines grew by 12.5 percent a year.

The combination of benzodiazepines and opioid painkillers (see the next section for more on those medicines) poses significant risk to cognitive ability and to overall well-being: data show that combinations of benzos with opioids contribute to at least 30 percent of opioid-related deaths.

Benzodiazepines should be prescribed only rarely in

BENZODIAZEPINES

With this and other drug lists, I provide only the chemical or generic name. Multiple brand names of each may exist, but on any pill bottle or prescription, you should be able to find this generic/chemical name, along with the drug's brand name.

alprazolam	estazolam	midazolam
bretazenil	etizolam	nimetazepam
bromazepam	ethyl loflazepate	nitrazepam
brotizolam	flubromazepam	nordazepam
chlordiazepoxide	flunitrazepam	phenazepam
cinolazepam	flurazepam	pinazepam
clonazepam	flutoprazepam	prazepam
clorazepate	halazepam	premazepam
clotiazepam	ketazolam	pyrazolam
cloxazolam	loprazolam	quazepam
delorazepam	lorazepam	temazepam
diazepam	lormetazepam	tetrazepam
diclazepam	medazepam	triazolam

older adults, in my judgment, and then, only for short periods of time. Because older people's bodies take longer to process these medications, the amount of active drug may build up. This, in turn, increases risk with these medicines not only of memory loss, but also of falls, fractures, and car accidents. People on benzodiazepines are more likely to visit the emergency room; elderly people who use them have a heightened risk of falls.

Withdrawal from benzos can lead to very serious side

effects. Addiction is a significant possibility with these medicines. Never try to kick them without supportive guidance from a healthcare professional.

Rising use of these drugs correlates with a steep rise in the diagnosis of anxiety disorders and insomnia in Western nations. People over age forty seem especially at risk. Fortunately, many natural alternatives exist for these issues: the herbal supplements theanine (found in green tea), valerian, passionflower, rhodiola, hops, ashwagandha, holy basil, kava, lemon balm, and chamomile; a substance called 5-HTP, which is made from the amino acid tryptophan; and omega-3 oils from fish or krill (tiny shrimp). The mineral magnesium has relaxant properties. Daily exercise—at least twenty minutes per day—will do a lot to reduce anxiety. Yoga, meditation, or slow, meditative martial arts forms like tai chi and chi kung are some of your best friends in reducing your need for antianxiety drugs. Leaning on supportive friends and family or seeking out skilled psychological coaching or therapy can also help you reduce any need for benzodiazepine drugs.

NARCOTIC PAINKILLERS (OPIOID ANALGESICS)

These medications are nervous system depressants used to relieve moderate to severe chronic pain. They calm the nervous system as well—an important part of helping people who are dealing with intractable pain, which can (of course) cause significant anxiety and interfere with sleep.

Narcotic painkillers contribute to many deaths each year, due to overdose or toxic combinations with drugs that also depress the nervous system. The pain signals blocked by these drugs, as well as the signals that move through the nervous system to elicit a feeling of anxiety,

OPIOID ANALGESICS

fentanyl	hydromorphone	oxycodone
hydrocodone	morphine	

involve chemical messengers that are needed for clear thought and good memory. We can't block these messengers without negatively impacting cognitive function.

Very serious pain may need this kind of serious pharmaceutical therapy, but if you and your doctor decide that its risks outweigh its benefits, nonsteroidal anti-inflammatory drugs (NSAIDs) may be a reasonable alternative. However, NSAIDs are less workable for people older than age fifty, who have a higher risk of gastrointestinal bleeding with those medicines. If pain is caused by rheumatoid arthritis or other autoimmune conditions, know that alternative medicine practitioners can help reduce pain with dietary, nutritional, and lifestyle programs.

CHOLESTEROL-LOWERING DRUGS (STATINS)

These drugs are used to lower cholesterol counts in people whose levels are judged high enough to increase risk of heart attack or stroke. Use of these medications in adults aged eighteen to sixty-four increased more than sixfold from 1988 through 1994.

Numerous studies show that statin drugs impair cognitive function. One 2009 study published in the journal *Pharmacotherapy* found that three of four people taking them had adverse cognitive effects that were linked to the medication. Ninety percent of these patients experienced demonstrable improvements in cognition—sometimes in only a matter of days—after statin use was stopped. Since 2012, the FDA has required a labeling statement on statin drugs about potential impacts on memory and cognitive function.

When we consider the role of cholesterol in the workings of the body, this makes perfect sense. Cholesterol is a vital building block for hormones and nerve cells. The brain contains one-fourth of the body's cholesterol! In particular, cholesterol is needed to foster connectivity between the cells that make up the nervous system. When we tamper with the body's mechanisms for producing cholesterol and deplete brain levels of this substance, we directly impact nervous system function. More recent research correlates statin use with lowered levels of a body chemical called leptin; low leptin is, in turn, correlated with a higher risk of Alzheimer's disease.

STATIN DRUGS

atorvastatin	lovastatin	rosuvastatin
fluvastatin	pravastatin	simvastatin

More and more Americans are being placed on statin drugs as prescribing guidelines shift. According to data from 2010, half of men and 36 percent of women aged sixty-five to seventy-four take statin drugs. Overall, one in four people over the age of forty-five take statins! The general notion is that these drugs carry little risk and that it's always best to keep cholesterol as low as possible. I could write an entire book about just how crazy this is—how oversimplified is modern medicine's attitude toward cholesterol counts and heart disease prevention—but for now, suffice it to say that there are probably millions of people taking these drugs and experiencing cloudy thinking and memory loss when they don't even really require the medication in the first place. If you are interested in natural ways to reduce cholesterol, Chapter 2 of this book will guide you in terms of a healthful diet that tends to lower cholesterol as a natural "side effect."

Eating fewer saturated fats and more olive oil, adding fiber from oats, barley, and vegetables and fruits, and taking fish oil supplements (1,000 to 3,000 milligrams (mg)/day) will give you a good start. Sublingual vitamin B_{12} (1,000 micrograms [mcg]) plus folic acid (800 mcg) plus vitamin B_6 (200 mg) daily can help keep cholesterol counts in balance. Exercise is one of the best ways to raise "good" high-density lipoprotein (HDL) cholesterol, which gives you more leeway in terms of your low-density lipoprotein (LDL) cholesterol. (What matters is the ratio between HDL and LDL, not the individual numbers.)

ANTISEIZURE DRUGS

This class of drugs was once used only to treat seizures, which are most often caused by epilepsy. But as has happened with so many medications, there's been a significant amount of cross-condition "creep" in their usage. Today, they're used to treat bipolar disorder and other mood disorders, mania, and nerve pain. Between 1999 and 2009, use of these medications nearly doubled in the United States, from 3.1 percent of the total population to 5 percent—about 15.2 million people.

The memory-dampening impact of these drugs has to do with their mode of action. They prevent seizures by suppressing signals that move within the central nervous system. Any drug that depresses the movement of signals

ANTISEIZURE DRUGS

acetazolamide	lamotrigine	rufinamide
carbamazepine	levitiracetam	topiramate
ezogabine	oxcarbazepine	valproic acid
gabapentin	pregabalin	zonisamide

in the brain is likely to also reduce ability to think and remember.

People with epilepsy may be able to switch to a drug called phenytoin, which seems to have less impact on memory than the drugs listed above. Chronic nerve pain treated with antiseizure meds may also respond to an antidepressant called venlafaxine, which may help clearer thinking prevail.

If mood disorders, bipolar disorder, or mania are the issues being treated, these have been shown to respond well to natural therapies, in particular high-dose fish oil. Most people in treatment for these issues end up switching their medications around periodically as their brains adjust and the medicine becomes less effective or causes more side effects. If memory loss and/or foggy thinking are issues with these drugs, talk to your doctor about ways to work with alternative medicines, natural therapies, talk therapy, or a combination of treatment approaches.

TRICYCLIC ANTIDEPRESSANTS

Tricyclic antidepressants (TCAs) are older medications— the first antidepressants developed, in fact, back in the 1950s. Newer antidepressants have largely replaced them, but they are still prescribed in some cases of depression that don't respond to newer drugs. They are also prescribed for anxiety disorders, eating disorders, obsessive-compulsive disorder, and chronic pain, and are also used to support people who are attempting to quit smoking. Women with severe menstrual cramps and hot flashes may also be prescribed these medications, which work by blocking the binding of neurotransmitters to receptors.

Among adults using TCAs, about 35 percent report some memory impairment. About 54 percent report difficulty with concentration. Lowering the dose or switching to more modern, more selectively acting antidepressants—selective serotonin reuptake inhibitors (SSRIs) or selective norepinephrine reuptake inhibitors (SNRIs)—can help restore better memory and thinking ability.

An important note: depression itself should not go untreated. It can be a serious issue that interferes with relationships, work, and overall quality of life. In addition, depression is a risk for cognitive decline and for Alzheimer's disease. The more intense the depression, the higher the risk of cognitive decline.

Now, this may bring up fear and frustration for those who believe the party line that depression is strictly a biochemical issue, something that strikes certain people and

TRICYCLIC ANTIDEPRESSANTS

amitriptyline	desipramine	protriptyline
amitryptilinoxide	doxepin	trimipramine
amoxapine	imipramine	
clomipramine	nortriptyline	

that is a chronic and largely incurable—if sometimes manageable—condition. That's another point I could go on about for roughly 100 pages, and this isn't the space or the time for that. For now, let me assure you that in most cases of depression, cure is possible. You may have to go outside the box of what the mainstream says you need, but it is almost always available. Genetics are not destiny here. The interplay of "nature" (genetic inheritance and biological tendencies) and "nurture" (environment, learning, ways of talking to ourselves and relating to others, choices about self-care and spiritual practice) is much more complex than the peddlers of biopharmaceutical therapies would like you to believe.

PARKINSON'S DISEASE DRUGS (DOPAMINE AGONISTS)

Let me begin by saying that Parkinson's disease has to be treated, and that these medications are our best bet at this point in holding the symptoms of this progressive illness at bay. Difficulties with memory and cognition are relatively minor concerns for people coping with this illness. However, dopamine agonists are increasingly being prescribed for restless legs syndrome (RLS) and to people with certain kinds of pituitary tumors.

Parkinson's disease is characterized by a deterioration of the part of the brain that produces the neurotransmitter dopamine. These drugs work by activating signaling pathways for this neurotransmitter. When we impact those pathways, we also impact movement (especially fine motor control), motivation, the way pleasure is experienced, and learning and memory.

The drugs levodopa and carbidopa may be good alternatives to dopamine agonists for people with Parkinson's

DOPAMINE AGONISTS

apomorphine	pramipexole	ropinirole

disease. They convert to dopamine in the brain. Carbidopa is used with levodopa because it reduces side effects, especially nausea. For those taking dopamine agonists for restless legs syndrome, and who notice impacts on memory and thinking ability, try avoiding caffeine, alcohol, and nicotine. If you use antinausea drugs (prochlorperazine or metoclopramide), antipsychotic drugs (haloperidol or phenothiazine derivatives), antidepressants that raise active levels of serotonin in the body (SSRIs), or cold and allergy medicines that contain sedating antihistamines, you should know that these can cause RLS symptoms. Daily exercise, increased sexual activity (orgasm increases dopamine and other opiates in the body that have been shown to help relieve RLS!), drinking more water, using progressive relaxation exercises, and taking supplemental magnesium may all help relieve this uncomfortable and mysterious condition.

HYPERTENSION DRUGS (BETA-BLOCKERS)

These are some of the oldest drugs still commonly prescribed. They've stood the test of time and are overall pretty darned safe and effective for their usual indications: high blood pressure (the most common indication), congestive heart failure, abnormal heart rhythms, chest pain, and migraines.

Beta-blockers work to reduce blood pressure and heart rate by blocking the actions of what we call beta-adrenergic agonists: norepinephrine, epinephrine (aka adrenaline), and others. In reducing the activity of those messengers, we also reduce the transmission of messages throughout the nervous system, and that can slow things down enough in the brain to impact thinking ability and memory.

Calcium channel blockers, another type of blood pressure–lowering medication, are also quite safe, time-tested, and effective, and they tend to impact memory and thinking ability less. For those using beta-blockers to treat glaucoma, another drug called a carbonic anhydrase inhibitor may be a better bet.

BETA-BLOCKERS

atenolol	propranolol	(Any other drug with a chemical name that ends with "-lol.")
carvedilol	sotalol	
metoprolol	timolol	

Even the folks at the Mayo Clinic agree that lifestyle changes and nutrition can take the place of medications for managing blood pressure. A healthful diet, focused stress-reduction strategies (yoga, meditation, guided visualization, or spiritual practice), and regular moderate exercise are good foundations. Losing weight around your midsection, if it's accrued there beyond forty inches (for men) or thirty-five inches (for women), will help drop high blood pressure too. Reducing dietary salt, drinking alcohol only moderately if at all, cutting back on caffeine, and ensuring that you have supportive relationships with family and friends also will help keep blood pressure numbers below the threshold requiring medication.

Ironically enough, at least one study has found that beta-blockers prescribed for hypertension may help prevent Alzheimer's disease (AD). This may have to do with the role of hypertension in creating microinfarcts, or tiny strokes, that can reduce brain function and memory over time. Controlling high blood pressure is clearly integral to AD prevention. What the study did not spell out, however, was whether controlling high blood pressure without medications would have an equal effect. We do know that exercise and good nutrition help stave off both hypertension and AD.

SLEEPING AIDS (NONBENZODIAZEPINE SEDATIVE-HYPNOTICS)

Ambien, Lunesta, Sonata: the brand names have such a soothing, melodious ring. But these so-called "Z drugs," used to treat insomnia and mild anxiety, have some serious downsides. They can cause amnesia or cause people to behave very strangely while asleep. Sleepwalking? Yes—but also try sleep-eating, sleep-drinking, sleep-cooking, or sleep-driving. Ambien has been a rising problem in traffic stops; it's one of the top ten substances found in the bloodstreams of people who are arrested for traffic violations. There is a confirmed link between these dangerous behaviors and drugs like Ambien, with that drug leading the field as the most popular among those wielding pre-

NONBENZODIAZEPINE SEDATIVE-HYPNOTICS

eszopiclone (Lunesta)	zaleplon (Sonata)	zolpidem (Ambien)

scription pads (26.5 million prescriptions were written for this drug alone in this country in 2012). Packaging information must warn users of the possibility of these kinds of side effects. These drugs are particularly potent when combined with alcohol.

Although these medicines are molecularly distinct from benzodiazepines, they act on the same physiochemical pathways and alter activity of the same chemical messengers. Addiction, withdrawal, and loss of memory and cognitive function are all possibilities with ongoing use of these medications. If you are using these drugs and want to stop, please do so with guidance from your doctor, as withdrawal symptoms can be significant.

Getting enough sleep—good quality sleep—is an issue for many folks over the age of fifty. Following the natural cycles of light and dark in your waking and sleeping, refraining from caffeine after noon, not drinking too much alcohol (it might relax you to sleep, but it is likely to jolt you awake as it wears off in the middle of the night), and getting daily exercise will all help. Keep the bedroom dim and use it only for sleep and sex—no glowing screens in the *boudoir*. Even a small amount of light at night can disturb sleep. Use progressive relaxation or meditation techniques to help you relax in the evening if anxiety keeps you awake.

The best natural sleep aid, by far, is melatonin, a hormone made in the pineal gland in the brain. Supplementing in doses from 3 to 10 mg before bedtime can help reestablish healthy sleep patterns. Animal research even suggests that melatonin can help reduce the risk of age-related memory loss. It is an antioxidant that reduces the accumulation of oxidative byproducts in the body—and those byproducts are part of the plaques that form in people with Alzheimer's disease. At the moment, we don't know for sure that it is safe to use every day—there is some concern that supplying the hormone through a supplement could reduce the body's natural production—but using the supplement two or three nonconsecutive days per week is believed to be safe.

INCONTINENCE DRUGS (ANTICHOLINERGICS)

Anticholinergics are most often used to treat a condition variously known as "overactive bladder" and "urge incontinence"—a sudden, extreme urge to urinate that can mean not getting to the bathroom in time.

Drugs in this class work by blocking the action of a chemical messenger called acetylcholine, which (among many other things) prevents involuntary contractions of muscles that control the flow of urine. The brain uses acetylcholine to activate learning and memory. In 2006, a study of oxybutynin (brand name Ditropan) found that using this drug impacts memory at a level comparable to about ten years of cognitive aging. The study's author said it this way: "We transformed these people from functioning like sixty-seven-year-olds to seventy-seven-year-olds." (Another oxybutynin product, Oxytrol for Women, is sold over the counter.)

Of all the drugs in this class, darifenacin (brand name Enablex) seems least likely to impair memory or cogni-

ANTICHOLINERGIC DRUGS

darifenacin	oxybutynin	tolterodine
mirabegron	solifenacin	trospium

tive ability; so, if you require an incontinence drug, see if you can get your physician to prescribe this one. Be sure your physician has ruled out any other possible reason for your urge incontinence: a bladder infection is one possible cause, and some medicines (blood pressure drugs, diuretics, or muscle relaxants) can cause side effects that resemble overactive bladder.

Once these are ruled out, I'd recommend trying some simple lifestyle changes, such as cutting back on caffeinated and alcoholic beverages, drinking less before bedtime, and doing Kegel exercises to strengthen the pelvic muscles that help control urination. As a last resort, try adult diapers, pads, or panty liners. As uncomfortable as these might make you, modern versions are thin and comfortable and give complete insurance against embarrassing accidents.

ANTIHISTAMINES (FIRST GENERATION)

The best known of these over-the-counter and prescription drugs is Benadryl (diphenhydramine). This medication was once the go-to remedy for allergy and cold symptoms, and its sedative effects are pronounced—as many parents will tell you, a little Benadryl is a handy thing for a child who's too sick to sleep. Antihistamines like these are also used to prevent dizziness, motion sickness, nausea, and vomiting. In rare cases, they have been recommended to help relieve anxiety or insomnia.

This class of drugs works by blocking the production of histamine, the chemical that causes allergic reactions. Unfortunately, the action of other body chemicals is blocked in the process, including that of chemical messengers/neurotransmitters called acetylcholine and serotonin. This reduces activity in centers where learning and memory happen. These medicines also appear to reduce the absorption of vitamin B_{12} in the stomach, and B_{12} is important for alertness and for good nervous system function.

FIRST-GENERATION ANTIHISTAMINES

brompheniramine	chlorpheniramine	diphenhydramine
carbinoxamine	clemastine	hydroxyzine

Today, these medicines are not often used to treat allergy symptoms, as nonsedating antihistamines like loratidine and cetirizine are available by prescription and over the counter. These nonsedating medicines are generally far better tolerated, especially for older adults.

The Mediterranean Diet: How Diet Can Impact Memory and Cognition

f I were to put my recommendations about what to eat to improve and preserve cognitive function in as brief a sentence as possible, I'd say, "Eat a Mediterranean diet."

THE MEDITERRANEAN DIET

The Mediterranean diet is comprised mostly of colorful vegetables (especially leafy greens); some fruit; lean protein (mostly fish, with some other meats—which the Mediterranean food pyramid places at the same level of consumption as sweets, meaning that they should be eaten rarely); some nuts and seeds (especially walnuts); whole grains; and dairy products in moderation, primarily as unsweetened yogurt and cheese. The diet is rich in legumes (beans), seeds, herbs, and spices; red wine is a hallmark of this diet as well. Refined sugar, unhealthy hydrogenated fats, fatty cuts of meat, butter, dishes dripping with cheese, and processed foods made with white flour do not make much of an appearance here.

The Mediterranean diet is the superstar of all health-promoting diets. It's got every ingredient known to help prevent or reverse all age-related conditions, from heart disease to type 2 diabetes to dementia—and yes, the risk of even some kinds of cancer can be reduced with adherence to a Mediterranean diet. A study involving over 1.5 million adults demonstrated that following this diet reduced the risk of death from heart disease and cancer, while also reducing the risk of Parkinson's and Alzheimer's diseases.

Based on all the available evidence about food as medicine to maintain mental sharpness and prevent Alzheimer's disease or other types of dementia, the Mediterranean diet appears to cover all the bases. Its preventive impact against stroke has recently been confirmed by a study of thousands of Spaniards, published in the vaunted *New England Journal of Medicine*. Ministrokes, also known as microstrokes, are known to be a major player in age-related damage to the brain that robs us of memory and cognitive ability, and if we can help prevent those with diet, we should. This diet will do just that.

That being said, let's look at a few important rationales for my recommendation, and a few points to be aware of in the specific quest to promote better brain function. What characteristics of the Mediterranean diet explain its positive impact on brain health and function? Here are the main points to recognize.

The Mediterranean Diet Is Anti-Inflammatory

The body has a delicately balanced set of mechanisms for fighting infection and healing injury. Inflammation is one part of that immune response. When you hurt a joint, it becomes hot, swollen, and painful as healing immune factors are drawn to the site. That's one kind of inflammation, and it usually resolves when the healing process is complete. A fever is a full-body inflammation that happens as the immune system launches an attack against a pathogen. Allergies and autoimmune diseases represent imbalanced inflammatory responses, and in those cases, inflammation does more harm than good. Modern diets and lifestyles (high stress, little physical activity, too little sleep, and diets that promote inflammation) create a state of low-grade, chronic inflammation in the body and the brain. Over time, this does damage to tissues that prematurely ages them and can set the stage for age-related conditions like dementia. Inflammation within blood vessel walls is a major contributor to stroke.

Our bodies make both inflammatory and anti-inflammatory chemicals. The foods we eat provide the building blocks for the making of those chemicals (primarily fats), and they impact the biochemical pathways that modulate inflammation. The upside of this is that inflammation can be impacted strongly through diet. The Mediterranean diet provides the body with potent nutritional factors—in particular, antioxidants and healthy fats—that have this anti-inflammatory effect.

The Mediterranean Diet Is High in Antioxidants

In Greece, where the Mediterranean diet is standard fare, people consume an average of six or more servings of antioxidant-rich, highly nutrient-dense vegetables and fruits each day. Their rates of dementia are lower than those in the United States (as are rates of the disease across central and eastern Europe: overall prevalence in the United States as of 2009 was about 6.5 percent of the population older than age sixty had some form of dementia—far ahead of the approximately 4.8 percent prevalence seen in those parts of Europe).

When the cells that make up our bodies metabolize fats, carbohydrates, or proteins to produce energy, they also produce a kind of "exhaust" known as free radicals. These submicroscopic particles can damage fats, proteins, and cholesterol. Our bodies have natural antioxidant defenses designed to "quench" these renegade particles, but we also need dietary antioxidants to maintain a healthy balance. High oxidative stress (chronically high, un-"quenched" free radicals) is linked to all kinds of outcomes no one wants, including most of the age-related diseases.

The brain is especially vulnerable to damage by free radicals. It is one of the most highly metabolic parts of the body—in other words, it uses more oxygen—and it also has low levels of antioxidant enzymes that are the body's natural protection against free radical damage.

Diets low in antioxidants are firmly linked to height-ened risk of dementia. Antioxidants are most abundantly found in nutrient-dense plant foods; in general, the more brightly colored the food, the higher the antioxidant con-tent. The Mediterranean diet is built mostly from these foods. Case closed.

HOW ABOUT SUPPLEMENTATION?

Supplementing antioxidants, anti-inflammatory factors, and other nutrients found in healthy foods may help support opti-mal brain function throughout life. I'm a big fan of nutrient supplementation, but it has to be done wisely, according to the latest research. At one time, it was standard practice to take megadoses of individual vitamins and minerals; today, we know a lot more about how to create a balanced intake of these nutrients without the potential long-term dangers of overdoing it or taking nutrients in the wrong balance. In Chap-ters 3 and 4, I'll go into depth about how to supplement with these factors to create additional antioxidant and anti-inflam-matory insurance against dementia and related issues.

The Mediterranean Diet Is Nutrient-Dense and Relatively Low in Calories

Animal studies have found that reducing caloric intake has much more than a slimming effect. Eating about a third less than one would naturally want to eat translates to the retardation of many aging processes; the delay of onset of most of the diseases associated with old age; and the lengthening of life span. Does this work for humans? Yes! Clinical trials investigating food restriction in healthy adults have shown significant drops in body weight, blood pressure, and blood sugars over periods ranging from two to fifteen years. This doesn't guarantee the dramatic impacts seen over the much shorter life spans of calorically restricted rats, but overall it looks like a very promising avenue for anyone interested in avoiding premature aging and loss of cognitive function.

The catch with the low-calorie diet is, of course, that eating this way could mean being hungry all the time. This has been found to cause no small amount of crankiness in those who attempt to restrict their caloric intake. And the best way to find middle ground here is to eat plenty of food, but to ensure that it is highly *nutrient-dense:* more nutrient bang for each caloric buck.

Whole foods rich in fiber and nutrients are inherently more satisfying than junk foods that are engineered to get you to eat much more of them than you need. Think of it this way: a head of broccoli is loaded with fiber and nutrients and only about 200 calories. A small bag of chips will have easily that many calories, much more fat, and a lot fewer antioxidant vitamins and minerals.

If you eat according to the dictates of the Mediterranean diet, your caloric intake will be well below what it would be if you ate a standard American diet. You won't need to worry about counting calories, and you'll still get all the benefits of a highly nutritious, low-calorie diet.

The Mediterranean Diet Is Low Glycemic

According to the American Diabetes Association, nearly 26 million American children and adults have diabetes; 79 million have prediabetes (a condition I'll explain more in a moment); and 1.9 million are diagnosed with diabetes each year. Most of these people are diagnosed with type 2 diabetes, also known as adult-onset diabetes—a form of diabetes created by an unhealthy diet high in refined carbohydrates and the overweight/obesity that often results from such a diet. Why does this information show up in a book about ways to preserve memory and cognition? Because type 2 diabetes is a major risk factor for Alzheimer's disease and other types of dementia.

Type 2 diabetes is diagnosed when a person's blood sugars stay too high over time. The cells lose sensitivity to the hormone insulin (a shift known as *insulin resistance*), which is supposed to move sugars from the bloodstream into the cells to be "burned" as fuel. High blood sugar is damaging to the body in many ways: it creates greater oxidative stress (more free radicals), accelerates inflammation, and directly damages the walls of arteries. The pancreas produces more and more insulin to try to overcome insulin resistance; this is also an unhealthy situation, since insulin in too-high concentrations is harmful to the insides of blood vessels. In prediabetes, insulin resistance has begun and sugars have started to rise, but they are below the threshold of a diabetes diagnosis. Still, microscopic damage to blood vessels is happening, particularly if antioxidant intake is low—a setup for potential strokes or heart attacks later on.

Type 2 diabetes and prediabetes both create excess inflammation and free radicals, both of which are bad news for brain function. Fortunately, these conditions both respond very well to changes in diet and lifestyle that reduce excess pounds and bring lots of nutrient-dense whole foods into the body. The Mediterranean diet is a great fit for this. It is *low glycemic,* which means the foods it contains do not create the blood sugar peaks and valleys that set the stage for prediabetes and diabetes.

Someone who is working to reduce blood sugars can modify the Mediterranean diet to eliminate any higher-glycemic foods. White bread, pasta, potatoes, and all but a few fruits (low-glycemic fruits include apples, stone fruits, cherries, and blueberries) can behave a lot like sugars in the body, and should be avoided by those with diabetes.

The Mediterranean Diet Is Made Up of Whole Foods, Especially Vegetables

The research is conclusive: a diet rich in vegetables—about as much as one would consume in the Mediterranean diet—reduces risk of dementia. Fruit is okay in small amounts here, but vegetables are the real key. Fruit is high in sugars, which can be an issue. I'll say more about that later in this chapter.

A vegetarian or vegan (no eggs or dairy) diet has been found to reduce risk of dementia. One study involving nearly 2,300 California residents found that those who ate any meat at all—including poultry and fish—were more than twice as likely to develop dementia than those who were vegetarians. When past meat consumption was factored in, the difference in risk widened even further, demonstrating a nearly threefold increase in risk for those who had been long-term meat-eaters. That's a pretty enormous difference in risk profiles, and worth noticing. Vegetarianism and veganism appear to be more protective for men than for women. Most other studies comparing vegetarian to high-meat diets demonstrate protective effects against dementia.

Most likely, the key factor in the vegetarian diet is the abundance of vegetables, fruits, whole grains, beans, nuts, and other foods that bring protective vitamins, minerals, phytochemicals, fats, and other compounds into the body. If you want to enjoy a few chunks of chicken, a filet of salmon, or even some range-raised, grass-fed beef with your abundant plate of plant foods, there is little chance that this will get in the way of the protective effects of those vegetarian delicacies. If you are consuming plenty of vegetables, it's fine to enjoy small servings of meat, dairy, or egg thrown in, if that helps you make the whole thing more satiating and delicious. Of course, if you're willing to try being vegetarian, you'll be going one step further to protect your health as you age.

The Mediterranean Diet Is Very Low in Refined Sugars and White Flour

The Mediterranean diet emphasizes whole grains and contains very little refined sugar. For our purposes, sugars and white flour are the same: they are rapidly metabolized and cause blood sugars to spike. A surge of insulin from the pancreas drops those blood sugars back down—sometimes so quickly that low blood sugar (hypoglycemia) results. Next comes a craving for more sugars or refined carbohydrates, and the cycle begins anew. Even mild hypoglycemia can make a person absentminded, forgetful, and spacey. Over time, being in this cycle sets the stage for insulin resistance and type 2 diabetes.

This cycle has the impact of accelerating inflammation, creating extra free radicals, and causing *glycation*: a binding of sugars to proteins that stiffens and ages tissues before their time. Chronic consumption of sugars and white flour crowds out other more nutritious foods from the diet, too, robbing the body of vital nutrients potentially supportive of good brain function. Go easy on the grains and choose whole versions—brown rice, whole barley, sprouted-grain breads and crackers—and avoid sugar as much as possible. You'll find you won't crave it after going cold turkey for a few days.

How about artificial sweeteners? Avoid them like the plague. Shifting your diet away from sweet tastes will only help you appreciate the more refined flavors of healthier foods. Aspartame, one of the more commonly used artificial sweeteners, has been found to be an *excitotoxin*, a substance that overstimulates neurons (nerve and brain cells), exciting them literally to death. The jury's still out on the safety of these fake sugars, so avoid them. One exception is a plant-derived sweetener called stevia, which seems to be fine when consumed in moderation.

The Mediterranean Diet Is Very Low in Trans Fats

Trans-fats are oils made solid and shelf-stable through a process called hydrogenation. The food industry thought of this as a good plan, but it turns out that these fats that industry built are among the most toxic fats around. They accelerate the inflammation we know to be bad for the circulatory system and bad for the brain.

The evidence that trans fats are dangerous is strong enough that the U.S. government created stricter labeling practices for processed food makers, but they can still use these fats and say the product contains 0 grams per serving if they keep it to below half a gram per serving. My suggestion is to avoid all foods that include hydrogenated or partially hydrogenated oils in their list of ingredients.

The Mediterranean Diet Is Rich in Polyunsaturated and Monounsaturated Fats, Especially Omega-3 Fats

Where trans fats accelerate inflammation, the Mediterranean diet is especially rich in anti-inflammatory fats and neutral fats. Omega-3 fats are found in fatty fish like salmon, mackerel, sardines, and anchovies, and most experts agree that it's a good idea to include fish in your diet two to three times a week. Hundreds of research studies have been published supporting omega-3s' preventive impact against heart disease, stroke, and some kinds of cancer.

Tuna is an acceptable source, but please stick with chunk light tuna, which is higher in fat and is less likely to contain high levels of neurotoxic mercury. Freshwater fish are likely to contain higher levels of mercury as well—not something you want to consume if you're concerned about the health and function of your gray matter.

Oats and other whole grains are rich in certain kinds of omega-6 fats that are also anti-inflammatory when incorporated into an overall healthy diet. Eating lots of sugars and refined grains can actually make these good fats pro-inflammatory, however, due to some complexities of the biochemical cascade that these fats go through at the cellular level.

Anyone who's been paying attention to the health news knows that olive oil is a clear winner in terms of healthfulness. The Mediterranean diet was the one that brought this oil into the world's cuisine, and for this, we should all be thankful.

A diet that contains moderate amounts of healthy fats

is more satiating. Healthful oils in the diet nourish the skin and nerve cells—in fact, research demonstrates that omega-3s are vital for maintaining or improving nervous system function (more on that in Chapter 4) and that supplementation may be a good idea for virtually everyone who plans to live to a ripe old age with their minds and memories intact.

The Mediterranean Diet Is Rich in Both Soluble and Insoluble Fibers and Plant Sterols

Soluble fiber and insoluble fiber, both found abundantly in whole grains, beans, vegetables, and fruit, each have their own roles in reducing the risk of age-related disease. Soluble fiber reduces the absorption of cholesterol into the body by binding its precursors in the gastrointestinal tract. Insoluble fiber improves bowel function, which helps reduce the body's reabsorption of toxins from the contents of the bowel. Plant sterols also block cholesterol absorption. They are found in healthy whole foods, including apples, grapes, and strawberries, and they are increasingly found as supplements in processed foods like buttery spreads. Getting adequate amounts of these fibers can reduce cholesterol counts by up to 5 percent.

The question that hasn't been answered is whether reducing cholesterol will help prevent dementia. There's definitely not adequate research support for reducing dementia using statin drugs. The majority of human data on blood and brain cholesterol counts does not support a role for cholesterol in causing Alzheimer's disease (AD). Some studies show that lowering cholesterol with medication helps with prevention, but others show no effect. One study found that older adults who had higher LDL ("bad") cholesterol and lower HDL ("good") cholesterol had slightly greater beta-amyloid deposits in their brains. This study made big headlines, but it didn't necessarily provide support for the use of statins as preventives against AD.

Here's why. Beta-amyloid deposits are characteristic of AD, but what's now being recognized—after decades of trying to target and prevent AD by reducing beta-amyloid—is that accumulation of this substance may just as easily be an *effect* of AD as a cause. And some research even shows *less* cognitive decline with higher beta-amyloid levels in people with AD. Some forward-thinking investigators even think it may be an antioxidant that accumulates because the brain is trying to knock out an unwanted invader, and that the invader—potentially a virus—is actually the root cause.

Now, this is definitely not license to mainline butter, bacon, and pork rinds, because a diet high in cholesterol is not so great for the body for other reasons. Foods very high in cholesterol also tend to be high in other things we don't want in our bodies (saturated fat, toxic chemicals that concentrate most highly in fatty foods) and tend to be missing the factors that most aid prevention.

A FEW SPECIAL DIETARY TIPS FOR GREAT COGNITIVE FUNCTION

To round out your new dietary adventure, consider a few specific do's and don'ts that aren't part of the Mediterranean diet, but that research suggests are important for maintaining good cognitive function as we age:

Do:

Eat lots of brain-healthy "superfoods." Walnuts, asparagus, blackcurrants, blueberries, fatty fish, ground flaxseed, kale, pumpkin seeds, radishes, red cabbage, spinach, summer squash, sweet potatoes, walnuts, watermelon: all these foods are high in B vitamins, which makes them brain-friendly dietary choices. Blueberries are particularly good for the nervous system, in that they contain a compound that prolongs neuron (nerve cell) life.

Try an exotic mushroom. Lion's mane mushroom, which research has found to improve neuronal proteins and the entire process the body uses to build nerve cells, can be found in health food and gourmet stores, or can be taken as a nutritional supplement. This superfood also seems to have a positive impact on mood and well-being.

Consume coconut oil. Rich in medium-chain triglycerides (MCTs), coconut oil can be your second go-to oil for cooking, after olive oil. Research suggests that MCTs are not readily stored as fat and that they are easily burned to produce energy. They are metabolized to end products called *ketone bodies,* which provide an alternative energy source for neurons. Some research suggests that in people with mild to moderate AD, MCTs improve cognitive ability.

Don't:

Eat lots of gluten-containing foods. Gluten is the major protein in wheat. Minimizing or even eliminating this substance in your diet is likely to score you big gains in brain function. For people who have difficulty digesting gluten—those with celiac disease—quitting wheat entirely has been found to drastically improve cognitive function and lift brain fog. The jury is out in terms of solid research for those who aren't diagnosed with celiac disease, but anecdotally, I can tell you that I've known a great many people whose thinking, memory, and attention, as well as their overall energy, took a big leap in a positive direction when they tried a gluten-free diet, and they noticed a big backward leap when they tried eating gluten again.

Load up on nonfermented soy. While fermented soy in the forms of miso and tempeh are healthy for the body as part of an overall balanced diet, non-fermented soy foods (including soymilk, tofu, and texturized soy protein) have multiple effects on the body that may contribute to foggy thinking. Fermentation transforms soy from a thyroid-hormone-blocking, digestion-disrupting, mineral-depleting food into a healthy and easily digested food. Reducing thyroid action and disrupting the absorption and action of vital nutrients is one sure way to diminish your ability to remember, attend, and learn! It's okay to consume non-fermented soy in moderation—a cup of soymilk here or a salad with baked tofu there is not going to make or break you—but these are not foods to eat every day.

Load up on foods high in fructose (fruit sugars). The research on this one is pretty conclusive: high dietary fructose—the main source for most modern Americans being high fructose corn syrup in sweetened processed food and drinks—is very, very bad for the brain. Dense doses of fructose have increased drastically in our diets, and that increase correlates with the similarly dramatic rise in obesity and type 2 diabetes. Both these conditions are associated with lower cognitive performance, cognitive decline, and dementia. Avoid any food sweetened with fructose and go easy on the fruit; emphasize fresh vegetables instead.

For more information, log onto www.nowfoods.com/
RememBrain-60veg-capsules.htm

3

Vitamin, Mineral, and Herbal Supplements for Better Brain Function

Nutritional supplements can be useful allies in the fight against memory loss and cognitive dysfunction. Only a few are adequately research-supported to merit inclusion here. In this chapter, we'll address vitamins and herbs with a strong research foundation as memory boosters: curcumin, ginkgo, bacopa, and vitamins D and B_{12}. In Chapter 4, we'll look at some other nutrient supplements with promise in this area: Huperzine A, Alpha-GPC, omega-3 fats, coenzyme Q10, and resveratrol.

CURCUMIN

Curcumin is a plant chemical found in the root of a plant called turmeric. It's best known as a part of curry powder. The root itself looks a lot like gingerroot on its exterior and is bright yellow on the inside. It has been part of Southeast Asian, Chinese, and Indian cuisine since antiquity, but over the last half century, it has also garnered substantial interest in research circles for its medicinal properties.

Turmeric is a staple spice in Asian Indian cuisine. Population studies show that there is less Alzheimer's disease (AD) in this population: countries with long-term consumption of curcumin show a 4.4-fold lower incidence rate of AD compared to the United States.

In animal studies, researchers have been able to reverse damage done to the brain with toxins, oxygen deprivation, or diets high in saturated fat or sugar with curcumin supplementation. These benefits don't only show up molecularly; the benefit shows up when animals are given memory tasks or put through mazes.

Curcumin impacts nearly all the biochemical pathways involved in age-related neurological diseases. It is:

- Anti-inflammatory: Curcumin impacts the process of chronic, low-grade inflammation at several key points.

- Antioxidant: Remember that the brain is more highly metabolic than the rest of the body and that it's low in antioxidant enzymes, which makes it more vulnerable to damage from free radicals. This damage is linked to AD and other forms of age-related memory loss. Animal research demonstrates that turmeric supplementation lowers measures of brain free-radical damage. Both test-tube and animal studies have found that curcumin inhibits the development of beta-amyloid plaques, the hallmark of AD; it's believed that this has to do with its antioxidant properties. Research shows that curcumin directly reduces levels of free radicals within cells.

- Antidiabetic: Curcumin has been found to support good blood sugar control and helps protect insulin-producing pancreatic beta cells from being destroyed.

- Neuroprotective: Curcumin positively affects several molecular pathways related to the building and maintenance of nerve cells.

- Longevity-enhancing: Recent research finds that curcumin enhances levels of a chemical called sirtuin-1 in rats. This chemical is linked to enhanced longevity. Other studies find that curcumin helps "guard" DNA in a way that may prolong cellular life span.

- Curcumin helps protect the cardiovascular system against the oxidative, inflammatory damage that leads to heart attacks and strokes. As if this weren't enough to recommend it, curcumin is also anti-mutagenic (it helps prevent DNA mutations that can be the beginnings of cancer) and anti-bacterial. It suppresses a body chemical called NF-kappa B (NFkB) that is needed for tumor formation.

Curcumin is a fat-soluble compound, so it's best to consume it in combination with fat. Some supplements deliver curcumin in combination with fats. In traditional cuisines, it's added to foods rich in fats. Piperine, the active constituent of black pepper, also helps absorption—one study found a twentyfold increase in absorption of curcumin with this nutrient combination.

Look for a curcumin supplement that contains at least 665 mg total curcuminoids, including curcumin, demethoxycurcumin, and bisdemethoxycurcumin. If it does not contain fats to enhance absorption, take it with a fat-containing meal or fatty acid supplements. Certain specialized curcumin extracts are crafted by supplement makers to have greater bioavailability—they are more efficiently absorbed and utilized by the body. One such curcumin extract is Longvida®, which has been shown to cross the blood-brain barrier more effectively than regular curcumin. Clinical studies using Longvida have shown great promise for affecting amyloid plaque in the brain and improving cognitive function.

GINKGO BILOBA

This beautiful tree is a source of plant medicine with a very long history of use in Chinese and Japanese medical traditions. It contains specific versions of plant chemicals called *flavonoids* and *terpenoids* that have been widely researched for their impact on cognitive function.

Studies on healthy subjects find that ginkgo is a good choice for general boosting of alertness when needed—for studying, or doing well on a test, or giving a presentation. One study of 188 healthy subjects aged forty-five to fifty-six found that 240 mg of a ginkgo extract called EGb 761 once a day showed significant improvements in quantity of recall (as measured by the number of correctly recalled appointments) compared to a placebo group that got an inactive pill instead of the supplement. Subjects that got the EGb 761 also had better results on other tests measuring recall and the ability to recognize a driving route. Brain scans found that ginkgo changed the brain blood flow patterns of middle-aged women to more closely resemble those of younger adults.

Other research supports its use in cognitively impaired people as well; ginkgo is, in fact, one of the most investigated supplements for cognitive disorders.

If you are using anticonvulsants, antidepressants, blood thinners or antihypertension drugs, know that these medicines can interact with ginkgo. Ginkgo can reduce the effectiveness of drugs like Tegretol (carbamazepine) and valproic acid (Depakote) and could cause a rare but serious side effect called serotonin syndrome when used with SSRI antidepressants like Prozac, Zoloft, Paxil, and Lexapro. Ginkgo may lower blood pressure, so using it with antihypertensives could lower blood pressure beyond a healthy level. And finally, ginkgo's blood-thinning effects can build on those of blood-thinning medicines like aspirin, Plavix, Ticlid, or Coumadin. Frequent use of Advil or other NSAIDs could create an adverse effect with ginkgo, since they both thin blood and could contribute to a dangerous bleeding-out if used together. Check with your pharmacist if any of these interactions seem possible for you.

Use a ginkgo supplement that contains a 50:1 standardized extract containing a minimum of 24 percent ginkgoflavonoglycosides and 6 percent terpene lactones.

BACOPA

Bacopa has a long history in Ayurvedic medicine, where it is known as *Brahmi* and is used to improve mental functioning and memory. A large-scale meta-analysis involving studies on 413 subjects shows that it improves cognitive ability, speed, and accuracy on tests of mental function over the course of about twelve weeks' use. It appears to be most valuable in improving retention of memories and information. Some studies support its use in reducing the impact of Alzheimer's disease, Parkinson's disease, and epilepsy.

Bacopa has antioxidant effects and inhibits the breakdown of acetylcholine, the neurotransmitter most important for memory. (Alzheimer's disease drugs target the same mechanism—the breakdown of acetylcholine.) This herb increases brain blood flow, reduces the buildup of beta-amyloid, and modulates the effects of the neurotransmitter dopamine, which impacts both mood and thinking ability. People who use this herb report improvements in mood.

Some evidence exists in favor of Bacopa as a remedy for digestive discomforts and for asthma (it helps relax airways). Use 300 to 450 mg per day, spreading the doses out in 150-mg increments from morning till night.

MAGNESIUM

According to Mark Hyman, M.D., a well-known natural health expert, a deficiency in magnesium makes you twice as likely to die earlier of heart disease than those who are not deficient in magnesium. It has so many important roles in the body that more than one scientific journal is devoted to publishing research about its uses in medicine. Tense, twitchy, or irritable muscles are likely to be deficient in magnesium. Insomnia, anxiety, irregular heartbeat, ADHD, asthma, irritable bowel, irritable bladder, and stomach reflux (a serious form of heartburn) are all, according to Dr. Hyman, suggestive of a lack of this important mineral. Deficiency is rampant, because this is a mineral found most abundantly in fresh, whole foods, especially sea vegetables, nuts, beans, and leafy greens—not the foods most of us eat enough of. Stress actually further depletes magnesium, creating a vicious cycle.

Anyone concerned about overall health and good cognitive function should supplement with magnesium. Take 400 to 2000 mg per day and choose a chelated version (magnesium bound to an amino acid to support better absorption)—magnesium L-threonate is a good choice. Taking nonchelated magnesium (for example, magnesium oxide) won't hurt you, but a lot of it will go right through your digestive tract without being absorbed. In fact, Milk of Magnesia, a tried and true noncramping laxative, is actually a solution of nonchelated magnesium.

VITAMIN D

This so-called vitamin is actually a hormone. It's produced in the skin during exposure to the sun, and is also found in food in small quantities. Lack of vitamin D is common, especially in places where there isn't a lot of sunshine. An enormous amount of research evidence supports a crucial role for vitamin D in the prevention of cancer, heart disease, osteoporosis, and Alzheimer's disease—most likely due to its anti-inflammatory and antioxidant actions.

Vitamin D has multiple nerve-fortifying and brain-protective impacts; animal studies show that deficiency can impair brain function, leading to negative changes in behavior. One study found that very low levels of vitamin D are predictive of fourfold the risk of cognitive impairments with aging. Very low D is also linked to a 1.6-fold increase in risk of Alzheimer's disease. The brain is loaded with vitamin D receptors and the most biologically active form of vitamin D has been found to help clear amyloid plaques in animal studies. In a rat model of prediabetes, vitamin D helped to both reduce inflammation and improve cognitive function.

Supplement with at least 1000 IU of vitamin D per day in the form of vitamin D_3 (cholecalciferol). If you don't get at least ten minutes per day of direct sunshine (or twenty to thirty minutes if you have dark skin), you may want to use more—up to 5,000 IU per day.

VITAMIN B_{12}

Deficiency of this vitamin is a well-known potential cause of slowed cognition, memory impairment, attention deficits, and dementia. B_{12} is needed to maintain and preserve the fatty myelin sheaths that cloak nerve cells and speed the conduction of nerve impulses. Deep deficiency can create symptoms of neurodegenerative disease due to damage to these myelin sheaths.

Commonly, processed foods are fortified with folate (B_2), another B vitamin. One Australian study found that in 1,354 subjects living in Australia between 2001 and 2011, people with low or normal blood vitamin B_{12} levels and high folate levels were more likely to have impairments in cognitive function than people who did not have high folate levels. It's not all that difficult to get too much folate if you consume a lot of fortified processed foods. This is another reason to avoid those foods and stick with fresh, natural, unprocessed fare wherever possible.

A deficiency of folate, B_{12}, and B_6 can lead to an imbalance called *hyperhomocysteinemia,* where levels of an amino acid called homocysteine build up in the bloodstream. The B vitamins are responsible for breaking homocysteine down into harmless byproducts; when B vitamins aren't present in adequate concentrations, homocysteine can build up to harmful levels that then cause damage to the delicate interior of blood vessels. Some evidence suggests that hyperhomocysteinemia is a risk factor for strokes—and remember that small strokes can be a major contributing factor to age-related memory loss—and heart attacks. One Chinese study found that supplementing people with high homocysteine with the right balance of B vitamins improved their cognitive function while reducing their blood homocysteine levels.

As we age, our bodies become less able to absorb B_{12} from food, so it's best to use a B_{12} supplement that is chewed or placed under the tongue to absorb directly into the bloodstream. Use a supplement that delivers a dosage of at least 1,000 micrograms (mcg) per day.

For more information, log on to
http://www.nowfoods.com/CurcuBrain-400-mg-
50-Veg-Capsules.htm

Brain
Supernutrients

The science of nutritional supplementation has come a very long way since my beginnings in this field. Where once we were limited to isolated vitamins and minerals as supplements to a healthy diet, we now know vastly more about how to use herbs and supernutrients to support optimal health. Much research has been done to enable us to understand the biological mechanisms that make these substances helpful for disease prevention, and supplement manufacturers are constantly improving delivery systems for these nutrients that increase their beneficial impact.

In this chapter, I'll inform you about a few of these supernutrients—those that seem most promising for maintaining and boosting great brain function.

HUPERZINE A

This supplement is derived from a type of Chinese club moss called *Huperzia serrata*. Like many of the other supplements I recommend for better brain function, it has antioxidant and anti-inflammatory effects; but it has a special impact on the body that makes it more promising than most as a natural therapy for Alzheimer's disease (AD): it works as a *cholinesterase inhibitor,* slowing the breakdown of a neurotransmitter called acetylcholine in the nervous system. Cholinesterase also happens to be the target of drugs prescribed to treat AD, a disease characterized by reduction in the activity of this important neurotransmitter.

Huperzine has been shown to improve cognitive function in AD patients and in patients with vascular dementia (VD)—dementia caused by multiple small strokes. A meta-analysis of studies involving 733 patients found that Huperzine A (Hup A) significantly improved scores on mental state and memory tests. Longer duration of use of this supplement led to greater effectiveness for AD patients. Animal studies suggest that Hup A is also useful for cognitive decline associated with diabetes; administering the supplements to rats with diabetes-associated cognitive deficits led to marked improvement on tests of memory function. What's more, these diabetic rats showed reductions in body weight when supplemented with Hup A.

Take this supplement in doses of no more than 400 mcg per day. It's best used in concert with other nutrients supportive of brain function. Try a product that combines Hup A with B_{12}, alpha-GPC, and phosphatidylserine (more on the latter two of these nutrients below).

ALPHA-GPC (L-ALPHA-GLYCERYLPHOSPHORYLCHOLINE)

Like Huperzine A, this supplement—derived from soy or other plants—inhibits the action of the cholinesterase enzyme, which breaks down the neurotransmitter acetylcholine. Alpha-GPC is naturally found in the brain, too; it's a substance the body uses to build nerve cells and to build acetylcholine. Studies show that alpha-GPC reliably boosts levels of acetylcholine in the brain, which will have a positive influence on thinking ability and memory.

When researchers administered this supplement to a type of rat specially bred to experience the same kind of age-related diseases we humans experience—type 2 diabetes, obesity, heart disease—their learning and memory capacity improved significantly. These rats started out with the rodent version of the age-related brain fog and forgetfulness that is so common in humans, and the supplement appeared to help reverse these changes.

Alpha-GPC is widely utilized as a prescription medication in Europe, where it is prescribed either to take as a pill or as an injection. It's prescribed for AD, but also for other kinds of dementia and to help people overcome damage caused by strokes. The United States hasn't quite gotten on that bandwagon yet, but you can get ahead of the curve by using this to supplement your healthy diet. It's appropriate also for healthy people who just want to improve memory, thinking, and learning skills.

Use 300 mg a day of alpha-GPC. Heartburn, headache, insomnia, dizziness, skin rash, or confusion have been reported with use of this supplement, but these are all minor and rare issues that reverse as soon as the supplement is stopped.

PHOSPHATIDYLSERINE (PS)

This is another nutrient derived from soy, but that also occurs naturally in the cells of the human nervous system—in fact, it's an essential part of all our body cells. It is a member of a class of compounds called *phospholipids*, and it helps build the permeable membranes that surround cells. Movement of nutrients into cells and pumping of wastes out of cells is one of the most fundamental functions for maintaining optimal health. Introducing PS into the body through supplementation may help this happen more smoothly and efficiently. In Scandinavia and Europe, PS is widely used to enhance memory and brain function.

A study of thirty volunteers aged fifty to ninety found that daily administration of 100 mg of PS for twelve weeks substantially improved memory recognition, memory recall, mental flexibility, and executive functions (mental processes that help to connect past experience with present action; used to plan, organize, strategize, remember, and attend to details, and manage time and space).

Phosphatidylserine appears most effective when used alongside omega-3 fatty acid supplements rich in DHA, a fatty acid that helps build optimally flexible, healthy cell membranes. One study found that when a combination of omega-3 and PS was given to eight elderly volunteers with memory complaints, a post-test revealed a 42 percent improved score on a test of word recall. I'll say more about omega-3s below, because they are excellent for the brain on their own merits. Blood pressure lowering may be a positive side effect of PS: in higher doses for longer periods, PS was found to lower blood pressure in elderly people with memory complaints.

Supplement PS in doses of 300 mg along with the other supplements recommended in this chapter.

OMEGA-3 FATTY ACIDS:
DHA (DOCOSAHEXAENOIC ACID) AND
EPA (EICOSAPENTAENOIC ACID)

The omega-3s EPA and DHA have made lots of health headlines in recent years for their protective effects against stroke, heart disease, cancer, inflammatory bowel disease, and autoimmune disease. Their roles in the body include blood clotting, taming excess inflammation, and the building of brain cell membranes.

Omega-3s have been studied as potential remedies for mood disorders, including bipolar disorder, ADHD, and depression, and much evidence supports their general positive effects on cognition and alertness. Some research suggests that higher concentration of DHA in the hippocampus of the brain correlates with improved memory. Adequate intake of omega-3s has been linked, in many studies, to reduced risk or incidence of cognitive decline and dementia. It is also associated with the decreased risk and incidence of several morbidities afflicting the elderly, including cognitive decline, dementia, rheumatoid arthritis, and macular degeneration.

One research team measured concentrations of brain omega-3s in postmenopausal women and then did brain scans to look at total brain volume and hippocampal volume. Eight years later, the women were rescanned, and those who started out with more omega-3 in their brains had greater volume by both measurements in the post-test. The researchers' conclusion: while normal aging results in overall brain atrophy, lower omega-3s may signal increased risk of hippocampal atrophy.

Some evidence points to a synergistic effect of DHA plus EPA, phospholipids like phosphatidylserine, and antioxidants like those described in previous chapters—not just for brain function, but for all the potential clinical applications of omega-3s. Modern diets tend to be low in this type of fat, which is found primarily in fish and other seafood. Marine animals get their omega-3s from marine algae; supplements with algae-sourced DHA are available for those who avoid fish. Certain kinds of omega-3 are found in oatmeal, flaxseeds, and walnuts. These foods contain a shorter-chain omega-3 called alpha-linolenic acid, or ALA, which is not as health-promoting as the longer-chain omega-3s from fish or marine algae: DHA (docosahexaenoic acid) and EPA (eicosapentaenoic acid). To have the benefits most supported by research, ALA has to be converted to long-chain DHA and/or EPA. Some bodies do this more efficiently than others. You're better off taking in the preformed long-chain omega-3s than counting on your body's ability to build them from ALA.

Aim to take in at least 500 mg per day of combined DHA and EPA in your nutritional supplement. Use a supplement made from salmon, anchovies, sardines, or krill (tiny shrimp eaten by larger fish and marine mammals), and be sure that it has been molecularly distilled to remove toxins like mercury, dioxins, and PCBs, which can concentrate in fish. Some brands label themselves "pharmaceutical grade," but there's actually no such thing as pharmaceutical grade fish oil. It's a standard that doesn't exist—just a meaningless bit of propaganda used by some manufacturers to try to make their products stand out.

COENZYME Q10 (UBIQUINOL)

Coenzyme Q10 (CoQ10) is part of most every cell in the body. It's an antioxidant that plays a vital role in the production of energy from the food we eat, while helping protect cells against free radical damage. Levels decline with aging—by some measures, this decline is in the neighborhood of 80 percent from youthful levels. Like many of the beneficial substances our body makes that also decrease with age, it appears linked to many of the age-related illnesses most of us would rather avoid. CoQ10 research shows that supplementing this nutrient may help counteract heart disease, diabetes, fatigue, and neurological issues like dementia.

Studies of aging mice supplemented with CoQ10 found that their proficiency in memory and spatial tasks improved. When researchers added CoQ10 to the Mediterranean diet, the diet's benefits seemed increased. CoQ10 helps the heart pump strongly and reduces irregular heart rhythms, which is associated with better overall circulation to the whole body—the brain included.

Remember from the chapter on prescriptions that can cause memory loss that statin drugs often create cloudy thinking and other cognitive challenges as well as a grinding level of fatigue. These side effects are believed to be due, at least in part, to a CoQ10-depleting effect of these medications. CoQ10 supplements can help reverse these problematic side effects.

Supplementation appears to be an effective way to reduce the impact of CoQ10 decline in the body. It is found in a few foods—mostly fish, meats, nuts, and oils, especially canola oil—but not in high enough concentrations to replicate the impact of supplementation. Most experts recommend 60 to 400 mg per day, with lower doses recommended for generally healthy people and doses of 200 mg and over reserved for those at risk for heart conditions.

RESVERATROL

If you enjoy red wine, you'll be happy to know that it contains a bounty of this particular antioxidant—one of the most-researched antioxidant compounds around. We know that resveratrol helps prevent heart disease and may also prevent some kinds of cancer; its impacts also seem to extend to brain health and function. Like curcumin, resveratrol may slow cognitive decline through some fancy impacts on cell function, including prevention of amyloid accumulation, modulation of the ways cells "talk" to each other, and effects on the longevity of DNA. Resveratrol appears to have a positive impact on specific proteins—sirtuins—that are known to be important for the prevention of neurodegeneration.

One positive impact of resveratrol is its blood glucose–lowering effect in type 2 diabetics. One study used it as an addition to medication in a group of sixty-six patients, and found that the nutrient had a substantial additive effect to the drug, increasing its blood pressure-lowering, blood glucose–lowering effects while also helping to lower insulin levels (a good thing in type 2 diabetes, where both blood sugars and insulin rise too high because insulin can't do its job anymore). It also reduces LDL and increases HDL. By now, you know that prediabetes and type 2 diabetes are major risk factors for Alzheimer's disease, and that controlling these disease processes through nutrition and nutritional therapy is crucial for protecting brain function.

Sipping a nice glass of red wine or eating red grapes will deliver resveratrol to your body, but if you are serious about preventing cognitive decline, you'll add it to your supplement regimen. Take 250 mg per day, and feel free to use a supplement that combines resveratrol with other powerful plant-derived antioxidants like grapeseed extract or green tea extract. A well-rounded array of antioxidants provides broad-spectrum protection; they work synergistically, replenishing each other as they are "spent" doing the work of quenching excess free radicals.

ACETYL L-CARNITINE

Amino acids are used by the body to build proteins. Sometimes, they also act as neurotransmitters. Carnitine has the special role of moving long-chain fatty acids like omega-3s into the parts of cells that produce energy (the mitochondria). Research published in the *American Journal of Clinical Nutrition* found that this nutrient significantly improved both physical and cognitive function in centenarians over a period of six months. If you add acetyl L-carnitine to your supplement program, use 500 mg per day. Expect a boost in both physical and mental energy.

DMAE (DIMETHYL-AMINO-ETHANOL)

This substance is made in the body. It's chemically similar to choline, and research dating back to the 1950s finds that as a supplement, it can be helpful for people who are depressed or experiencing mental decline. Brain scan studies of people who've taken a dose of DMAE show brain wave changes that specifically indicate greater alertness and focus.

Start with a low dose of 50 to 150 mg, because it can be very energizing and you won't want to take any more than absolutely needed. High doses can create irritability and tension.

5-HTP

This nutrient is produced during the breakdown of an amino acid called L-tryptophan. Supplements are usually made from an African plant called *Griffonia simplicifolia*. 5-HTP increases brain levels of the neurotransmitter serotonin, which plays important roles in sleep, appetite, mood, and pain sensitivity. In Europe, it is commonly used to treat depression. Do not use 5-HTP with any medication that impacts serotonin levels, including the SSRI and SNRI drugs commonly used to treat depression and anxiety disorders. If you decide to try this supplement, take 100 mg per day.

For more information, log onto www.nowfoods.com/RememBrain-60veg-capsules.htm

Stress, Sleep, Socializing, Exercise, Learning, and Your Brain

Aging is associated with progressive losses in function across multiple systems, including sensation, cognition, memory, motor control, and affect. The traditional view has been that functional decline in aging is unavoidable because it is a direct consequence of brain machinery wearing down over time. In recent years, an alternative perspective has emerged . . . Studies of adult brain plasticity have shown that substantial improvement in function and/ or recovery from losses in sensation, cognition, memory, motor control, and affect should be possible, using appropriately designed behavioral training paradigms.

—"Brain Plasticity and Functional Losses in the Aged: Scientific Bases for a Novel Intervention." Mahncke, H. W., Bronstone, A., and Merzenich, M. M. *Progress in Brain Research*, 2006,157:81–109.

You've probably heard that saying, "Biology is not destiny." Like most sayings we hear over and over again, this one is true, but complex. We may have genetic propensities toward age-related brain changes, and we may have lived our lives or fed our bodies in ways that have sped those changes up. However: What we can break down, we can build up again to some extent. We can do this through excellent dietary choices; through prudent nutritional supplementation (which we covered in Chapters 3 and 4); and through particular lifestyle shifts or emphases that are research-proven to promote better cognitive function and/or prevent dementia.

Your social interactions, your level of active learning and engagement, your level of physical activity, and the quality of your sleep can all make substantial differences in your ability to think, attend, and remember. Let's look at what the research has to say about this—you'll find it is every bit as compelling as any research about diet or nutritional supplements. Incorporating every part of this memory-boosting plan will be your very best bet at maintaining optimal brain function throughout your life.

THE IMPORTANCE OF SOCIAL CONNECTEDNESS

A very large meta-analysis—a type of study that entails combining the results of multiple smaller studies on the same topic—looked at the role of social connectedness and integration in health and life span. Over 300,000 total subjects were involved in the study. The investigators found that the risk associated with lacking this one factor was equivalent to the risk of smoking fifteen cigarettes a day; to being an alcoholic; and to being sedentary (not exercising). Although the health risks of obesity are all over the news these days, it's actually twice as harmful to be lonely and lack social connection.

When people are socially isolated, their risk of Alzheimer's disease roughly doubles; the risk of other kinds of dementia is higher as well. Loneliness correlates strongly with poorer cognitive function and with more rapid cognitive decline over time. This association is particularly strong for women, and the cognitive advantages of larger social networks are more protective for older women.

Protecting your cognitive function over time entails maintaining a good social network. Make this as much a priority as eating well, using nutritional supplements, and exercising.

PHYSICAL ACTIVITY AND BRAIN FUNCTION

In children, better fitness scores predict higher scores on tests of cognitive function. This link between physical and mental fitness doesn't disappear with the passing of time. In studies of aged mice, exercise has been found to have pro-cognitive effects. Human studies find that exercise—especially more intense exercise—benefits the aging brain. In one study, people with lower cardiorespiratory function had accelerated trajectories of cognitive decline over time. In other words, just strolling around the local shopping center at two miles per hour will not have the greatest benefit, but working out just hard enough to really feel yourself pushing, sweating, and breathing hard will.

A review of studies on cognitive function in women found that regular physical activity significantly slows both cognitive and physical decline. Women who exercised or had active lifestyles had lower overall risk of death during the course of the study.

Regular exercise at about 85 percent of maximum heart rate for one's age may be especially key for reducing Alzhemier's disease risk in people who are obese. Exercise is one of the best ways to prevent diabetes, which is a disease that accelerates all the factors known to contribute to dementia and loss of cognitive function (including inflammation, excess free radical formation, and poor blood vessel health). One study found that prediabetic obese people could slow the progression of fatty liver disease, which in turn is associated with a higher risk of dementia, with a relatively intense exercise regimen. Treadmill walking for an hour a day at this intensity level (i.e., 85% of maximum heart rate) raised levels of a hormone, *adiponectin,* which improves insulin responsiveness and reduces inflammation and free radical production throughout the body.

Mindfulness exercise modalities such as yoga also promote better brain function. They improve sleep quality, reduce anxiety, and enhance overall energy levels. Poor sleep and the constant grind of anxiety are both damaging to cognitive function; in fact, uncontrolled stress is used to induce cognitive decline in lab animals. A daily practice incorporating mindfulness and relaxing yoga sequences is a great investment in good lifelong brain function.

THE IMPORTANCE OF QUALITY SLEEP

Insomnia and aging can go hand in hand. As many as 40 percent of people over sixty experience insomnia, frequent waking, and disrupted sleep. Poor health and depression are commonly associated with poor sleep; so are problems sustaining attention, slower response time, and difficulty remembering. Studies show that sleep deprivation impairs neuronal connectivity in parts of the brain important in working memory.

In other words: if you think maybe you're having too many "senior moments," or if you worry that forgetfulness and difficulty sustaining attention might mean you're on your way to developing dementia, it may just be that you need more sleep or better quality sleep. Not only can lack of good sleep create foggy thinking and memory lapses; it also appears, over time, to contribute to the development of Alzheimer's disease. Amyloid-beta depositions in the brain have been found to parallel sleep deficits, and disruptions in *circadian rhythms* (adherence to cycles of sleep during dark and wakefulness during daylight) are a known risk factor for dementia.

So what's the best way to ensure eight hours a night of great sleep as we age? A few pointers:

- Ensure that your bed is adequately comfortable and your room as dark as possible during the nighttime hours. Even dim light at night reduces melatonin production in the brain, which in turn can disrupt sleep.

- Don't drink in the hour or so before bed, especially caffeinated drinks or alcohol. If you know you tend to snore, get evaluated for sleep apnea and get treatment if this is an issue for you.

- Avoid napping in late afternoon or evening, and keep naps to ten to twenty minutes or less when you do take them.

- Exercise in the daytime to enhance sleep at night.

- Learn relaxation and self-hypnosis techniques to improve your ability to relax when anxiety or tension interrupt sleep.

- Don't eat heavy meals or exercise after 5:00 P.M.

- Go to bed and rise at the same time every day, preferably in accordance with the rhythms of light and dark outside.

- Use valerian or passionflower, both relaxing herbs, or melatonin (0.25 to 3 mg, preferably taken under the tongue as a sublingual tablet) to bring on sleep where needed. Magnesium supplements can also help relax the body and bring on deeper sleep.

- If you do find yourself unable to sleep, don't stay in bed worrying about it. Get up and do something calm that doesn't require a lot of bright light: read a book, meditate, or listen to an audiobook, podcast, or soothing music.

STRESS AND SENIOR MOMENTS

We all know how stress impacts our ability to think and remember. Stress and anxiety knock us all down several IQ points by putting us in "fight-or-flight" mode, where we don't have easy access to the higher thinking parts of the brain. At some level, even if we're just anxious about forgetting someone's name or about remembering how to drive somewhere important, our bodies and brains believe that danger is afoot, and fighting, fleeing, or freezing trump calm, intelligent thoughtfulness.

Take stress relief seriously. Become aware of the signals your body gives you that it's stressed: Does your jaw clench? Do you get butterflies in your stomach? Do you get snappish with other people or harder on yourself? Develop coping mechanisms for those moments, and have an overall plan for self-care that includes reflection, some kind of contemplative practice like meditation, and plenty of lightness and laughter. Sometimes, a skilled therapist is the best ally for those who want to find better ways to cope with life's stresses. Some nutrients can be supplemented with relaxant effects—magnesium is one that's particularly valuable in this regard. Reducing or eliminating sugar and refined grains in your diet will help a lot as well. In a relaxed state, you'll find yourself eased into your higher brain centers, and with that will come easier access to memories and improved thinking ability.

USE IT OR LOSE IT:
KEEPING YOUR BRAIN TRAINED

To keep your brain young, stay involved in activities that stimulate your senses, challenge your cognitive abilities, get you moving in new ways, and run you through your full gamut of emotions. (Yes—it does appear that having a healthy range of emotions, and expressing them in a healthy way, helps cognitive function.) Studies show that choosing to engage in these kinds of activities keeps neural pathways engaged and may even forge some new ones.

This doesn't have to be overly challenging or time-consuming. Simply learning to use a new device—an iPad, for example, or a new smartphone—helps keep the brain firing on all cylinders and improves memory. Social interactivity, community activism, interesting relationships, taking a class, seeing good films, going to museums, and experimenting with new exercise modalities will all help support good memory and cognition with the passing of years. This isn't conjecture—the research shows it to be true.

It's never too early to start preventing memory loss through a rich menu of activities, learning, hobbies, and physical activity. Some research shows that a life spent engaged in these kinds of activities expands something called *cognitive reserve,* a storehouse of mental capacity and energy that extends the brain's healthy, high-functioning life span.

One especially interesting study published in 1988 described postmortem examinations of the brains of 137 elderly people. For those who had Alzheimer's disease (AD), there was a large discrepancy between the degree of pathology—the predominance of beta-amyloid and other signature changes with this disease—and the symptoms the people experienced while alive. In other words, some had extensive AD-related changes but no clinical signs of the disease. Those people had greater brain weights and more neurons than other people their age. The researchers believed that this might support the idea that when people begin with a greater cognitive reserve, they may have AD-related biological changes without the actual symptoms of the disease setting in!

Take-home: there is a clear connection between a lifestyle involving lots of learning, experimenting, curiosity, and emotion and greater cognitive reserve. Food for thought.

For more information, log onto www.nowfoods.com/ RememBrain-60veg-capsules.htm

Conclusion

It has been said before that "If you keep doing what you've been doing, you'll keep getting what you've been getting." By now, you understand that dementia and Alzheimer's disease are very serious conditions and diseases, and this book is about your doing something new that will change your brain health and memory for the better.

If your memory is not as sharp as it was when you were younger, you can't sit by and continue to do the same old things and expect different results. I feel that you, my reader, are now in a much better position to improve your memory and cognitive function by having read this book. You understand how certain vitamins, minerals, and herbal supplements can help your brain health. You also now have important information about which prescription drugs can cause memory loss and reduce cognitive function.

Take a proactive role in your brain health, memory, and overall wellness starting today. I wish you a super memory and optimal health in general.

Be well,
Dr. Earl Mindell

References

Introduction

Beck, M. (May 27, 2008). The science behind "senior moments." *Wall Street Journal* Online. http://online.wsj.com/article/SB121155964904517695.html

Gentile, JM. NIH embraces bold, 12-year scientific vision for BRAIN Initiative. http://www.huffingtonpost.com/news/brain-initiative/

Chapter One

Esteban S, Garau C, & Aparicio S. Chronic melatonin treatment and its precursor L-tryptophan improve the monoaminergic neurotransmission and related behavior in the aged rat brain. *J Pineal Res* 2010 Mar;48(2):170–177.

http://www.npr.org/blogs/health/2013/11/12/244815077/a-shift-in-cholesterol-advice-could-double-statin-use

Jaslow R. Beta blockers may stave off dementia, study suggests. CBS NEWS January 8, 2013, 2:57 PM. http://www.cbs news .com/news/beta-blockers-may-stave-off-dementia-study-suggests/

Kay GG & Ebinger U. Preserving cognitive function for patients with overactive bladder: evidence for a differential effect with darifenacin. *Int J Clin Pract.* Nov 2008; 62(11): 1792–1800.

Kay GG. The effects of antihistamines on cognition and performance. *J Allergy Clin Immunol* 2000 Jun;105(6 Pt 2): S622–627.

Knox R. A shift in cholesterol advice could double statin use. Nov 12, 2013. Source: American Heart Association and The American College of Cardiology

Lam JR, Schneider JL, Zhao W, et al. Proton pump inhibitor and histamine 2 receptor antagonist use and vitamin B12 deficiency. *Med Health Care Philos* 2007 Jun;10(2):141–151.

Lieb W, Beiser AS, Vasan RS, et al. Association of plasma leptin levels with incident Alzheimer disease and MRI measures of brain aging. *JAMA* 2009 Dec 16;302(23):2565–2572.

Mahowald MW. Disorders of sleep. In: Goldman L, Schafer AI, eds. *Cecil Medicine*. 24th ed. Philadelphia, Pa: Saunders Elsevier; 2011:chap 412.

Nonaka A, Masuda F, Nomura H, et al. Impairment of fear memory consolidation and expression by antihistamines. *Brain Res* 2013 Feb 1;1493:19–26.

PR Newswire. Prescriptions for benzodiazepines rising and risky when combined with opioids, Stanford researchers warn. http://www.prnewswire.com/news-releases/prescriptions-for-benzodiazepines-rising-and-risky-when-combined-with-opioids-stanford-researchers-warn-248920831.html

Stagnitti MN. Trends in anticonvulsants utilization and expenditures for the US civilian noninstitutionalized population, 1999 and 2009. June 2012. http://meps.ahrq.gov/mepsweb/data_files/ publications/st372/stat372.pdf

Sun YM, Luan Y, Wang LF, et al. Effect of statin therapy on leptin levels in patients with coronary heart disease. *Peptides* 2010 Jun;31(6):1205-7.

Van der Mussele S, Fransen E, Struyfs E, et al. Depression in mild cognitive impairment is associated with progression to

Alzheimer's disease: A longitudinal study. *J Alzheimers Dis* 2014 Jul 7.

Wehrwein P. Statin use is up, cholesterol levels are down: are Americans' hearts benefiting? Posted April 15, 2011 at Harvard Health site: http://www.health.harvard.edu/blog/statin-use-is-up-cholesterol-levels-are-down-are-americans-hearts-benefiting-201104151518

Yanai K, Rogala B, Chugh K, et al. Safety considerations in the management of allergic diseases: focus on antihistamines. *Curr Med Res Opin* 2012 Apr;28(4):623–642.

Chapter Two

DeFelice FG & Ferreira ST. Inflammation, defective insulin signaling, and mitochondrial dysfunction as common molecular denominators connecting type 2 diabetes to Alzheimer disease. *Diabetes* 2014 Jul;63(7):2262–2272.

Everitt AV, Hilmer SN, Brand-Miller JC, et al. Dietary approaches that delay age-related diseases. *Clin Interv Aging* Mar 2006; 1(1):11–31.

Giem P, Beeson WL, & Fraser GE. The incidence of dementia and intake of animal products: preliminary findings from the Adventist Health Study. *Neuroepidemiology* 1993;12(1):28–36.

Halliwell B & Gutteridge JM. The importance of free radicals and catalytic metal ions in human diseases. *Mol Aspects Med* 1985:8;89–193.

Lakhan S & Kirchgessner A. The emerging role of dietary fructose in obesity and cognitive decline. *Nutr J* 2013;12:114.

Lichtwark T, Newnham ED, Robinson SR, et al. Cognitive impairment in celiac disease improves on a gluten-free diet and correlates with histological and serological indices of disease severity. *Alimentary Pharmacology & Therapeutics* 2014.

Mediterranean diet: a heart-healthy eating plan. http://www .mayoclinic.org/healthy-living/nutrition-and-healthy-eating/ in-depth/mediterranean-diet/art-20047801

Sharma A, Bemis M, & Desilets AR. Role of medium chain triglycerides [Axona(R)] in the treatment of mild to moderate Alzheimer's disease. *Am J Alzheimers Dis Other Demen* 2014 Jan 9. (E-Pub Ahead of Printing)

Stamets P. Lion's mane: a mushroom that improves your memory and mood? http://www.huffingtonpost.com/paul-sta-mets /mushroom-memory_b_1725583.html

Umegaki H. Type 2 diabetes as a risk factor for cognitive impairment: current insights. *Clin Interv Aging* 2014 Jun 28; 9:1011–1019.

Chapter Three

Aguiar S & Borowski T. Neuropharmacological review of the nootropic herb *Bacopa monnieri. Rejuvenation Res.* 2013 Aug;16(4):313–326.

Anastasiou CA, Yannakoulia M, & Scarmeas N. Vitamin D and cognition: an update of the current evidence. *J Alzheimers Dis.* 2014 May 12.

Belviranli M, et al. Curcumin improves spatial memory and decreases oxidative damage in female rats. 2013 *Biogerontology* 14:187–196.

Briani C, Dalla Torre C, Citton V, et al. Cobalamin deficiency: clinical picture and radiological findings. *Nutrients.* 2013 Nov 15;5(11):4521–4539.

Canevelli M, Adali N, Kelaiditi E, et al. Effects of Gingko biloba supplementation in Alzheimer's disease patients receiving cholinesterase inhibitors: data from the ICTUS study. *Phytomedicine* 2014 May 15;21(6):888–892; ICTUS/DSA Group.

Cheng D, Kong H, Pang W, et al. B vitamin supplementation

improves cognitive function in the middle aged and elderly with hyperhomocysteinemia. *Nutr Neurosci* 2014; Jun 18.

Dickens AP, Lang IA, Langa KM, et al. Vitamin D, cognitive dysfunction and dementia in older adults. *CNS Drugs* 2011 Aug;25(8):629–639.

Durk MR, Han K, Chow EC, et al. 1alpha,25-Dihydroxyvitamin D3 reduces cerebral amyloid-beta accumulation and improves cognition in mouse models of Alzheimer's disease. *J Neurosci.* 2014 May 21;34(21):7091-10.

Ganguli M, Chandra V, Kamboh MI, et al. Apolipoprotein E polymorphism and Alzheimer's disease: the Indo-US cross-national dementia study. *Arch. Neurol.* 2000;57:824–830.

Hyman, Mark, Magnesium: The most powerful relaxation mineral available. http://www.huffingtonpost.com/dr-mark-hyman/magnesium-the-most-powerf_b_425499.html. May 20, 2010.

Kaschel R. Specific memory effects of Ginkgo biloba extract EGb 761 in middle-aged healthy volunteers. *Phytomedicine* 2011 Nov 15;18(14):1202–1207.

Kongkeaw C, Dolokthornsakul P, Thanarangsarit P, et al. Meta-analysis of randomized controlled trials on cognitive effects of *Bacopa monnieri* extract. *J Ethnopharmacol.* 2014 Jan 10;151(1):528–535.

Ledford H. Sirtuin protein linked to longevity in mammals. *Nature* 2012 Feb 22; http://www.nature.com/news/sirtuin-protein-linked-to-longevity-in-mammals-1.10074.

Lee WH, Loo CY, Bebawy M, et al. Curcumin and its derivatives: their application in neuropharmacology and neuroscience in the 21st century. *Curr Neuropharmacol* Jul 2013; 11(4):338–378.

Moore EM, Ames D, Mander AG, et al. Among vitamin B_{12} deficient older people, high folate levels are associated with worse cognitive function: combined data from three cohorts. *J Alzheimers Dis.* 2014;39(3):661–668.

Roodenrys S, Booth D, Bulzomi S, et al. Chronic effects of Brahmi (*Bacopa monnieri*) on human memory. *Neuropsychopharmacology.* 2002 Aug;27(2):279–281.

Sakatani K, Tanida M, Hirao N, et al. Gingko biloba extract improves working memory performance in middle-aged women: role of asymmetry of prefrontal cortex activity during a working memory task. *Adv Exp Med Biol.* 2014;812: 295–301.

Shoba G, Joy D, Joseph T, et al. Influence of piperine on the pharmacokinetics of curcumin in animals and human volunteers. *Planta Med* 1998 May;64(4):353–356.

Sikora E, Scapagnini M, & Barbagallo M. Curcumin, inflammation, ageing and age-related diseases. *Immun Ageing* 2010 Jan 17;7(1):1.

Soni M, Kos K, Lang IA, et al. Vitamin D and cognitive function. *Scand J Clin Lab Invest Suppl.* 2012 Apr;243:79–82.

Wu A, Ying Z, & Gomez-Pinilla F. The interplay between oxidative stress and brain-derived neurotrophic factor modulates the outcome of a saturated fat diet on synaptic plasticity and cognition. *Eur J Neurosci.* 2004 Apr;19(7):1699–1707.

Yong Zhang, DY. Leung, M, Brittany N, et al. Vitamin D inhibits monocyte/macrophage proinflammatory cytokine production by targeting mapk phosphatase-1. *Journal Immunol* 2012 March 1.

Chapter Four

Bauer I, Hughes M, Rowsell R, et al. Omega-3 supplementation improves cognition and modifies brain activation in young adults. *Hum Psychopharmacol.* 2014 Mar;29(2): 133–144.

Cao D, Kevala K, & Kim HY. Docosahexaenoic acid promotes hippocampal neuronal development and synaptic function. *J Neurochem* 2009 Aug 13.

Connor S, Tenorio G, Clandinin MT, et al. DHA supplementation enhances high-frequency, stimulation-induced synaptic transmission in mouse hippocampus. *Applied Physiology, Nutrition, and Metabolism* 2012 June 20.

Daiello LA, Gongvatana A, Dunsiger S, et al. Association of fish oil supplement use with preservation of brain volume and cognitive function. Alzheimer's Disease Neuroimaging Initiative. *Alzheimers Dement* 2014 Jun 18.

Danthiir V, Hosking D, Burns NR, et al. Cognitive performance in older adults is inversely associated with fish consumption but not erythrocyte membrane n-3 fatty acids. *J Nutr.* 2014 Mar;144(3):311–320.

Di Perri R, Coppola G, Ambrosio LA, et al. A multicenter trial to evaluate the efficacy and tolerability of alpha-glycerylphosphorylcholine versus cytosine diphosphocholine in patients with vascular dementia. *J Int Med Res.* 1991 Jul–Aug;19 (4):330–341.

Dimpfel W, Wedekind W, & Keplinger I. Efficacy of dimethylaminoethanol (DMAE) containing vitamin-mineral drug combination on EEG patterns in the presence of different emotional states. *Eur J Med Res* 2003 May;8(5):183–191.

Drago F, Mauceri F, Nardo L, et al. Behavioral effects of L-alpha-glycerylphosphorylcholine: Influence on cognitive mechanisms in the rat. *Pharmacol Biochem Behav.* 1992 Feb;41(2): 445–448.

Durk MR, Han K, Chow EC, et al. 1alpha,25-Dihydroxyvitamin d3 reduces cerebral amyloid-beta accumulation and improves cognition in mouse models of Alzheimer's disease. *J Neurosci.* 2014 May 21;34(21):7091–7101.

Erbas O, Solmaz V, Aksoy D, et al. Cholecalciferol (vitamin D 3) improves cognitive dysfunction and reduces inflammation in a rat fatty liver model of metabolic syndrome. *Life Sci* 2014 May 17;103(2):68–72.

Fratesi JA, Hogg RC, & Young-Newton GS. Direct quantitation of omega-3 fatty acid intake of Canadian residents of a long-term care facility. *Appl Physiol Neurol Metab.* 2009 Feb; 34(1):1–9.

Ha GT, Wong RK, & Zhang Y. Huperzine A as potential treatment of Alzheimer's disease: an assessment on chemistry, pharmacology, and clinical studies. *Chem Biodivers* 2011 Jul;8(7):1189–1204.

Kidd PM. Omega-3 DHA and EPA for cognition, behavior, and mood: clinical findings and structural-functional synergies with cell membrane phospholipids. *Altern Med Rev* 2007 Sep;12(3): 207–227.

Konagai C, Yanagimoto K, Hayamizu K, et al. Effects of krill oil containing n-3 polyunsaturated fatty acids in phospholipid form on human brain function: a randomized controlled trial in healthy elderly volunteers. *Clin Interv Aging.* 2013;8: 1247–1257.

Leckie RL, Manuck SB, Bhattacharjee N, et al. Omega-3 fatty acids moderate effects of physical activity on cognitive function. *Neuropsychologia.* 2014 Jul;59:103–11.

Malaguarnera M, Cammalleri L, Gargante MP, et al. L-carnitine treatment reduces severity of physical and mental fatigue and increases cognitive functions in centenarians: a randomized and controlled clinical trial. *Am J Clin Nutr* 2007; 86(6):1738–1744.

Mao XY, Cao DF, Li X, et al. Huperzine A ameliorates cognitive deficits in streptozotocin-induced diabetic rats. *Int J Mol Sci.* 2014 May 5;15(5):7667–7683.

Pottala JV, Yaffe K, Robinson JG, et al. Higher RBC EPA + DHA corresponds with larger total brain and hippocampal volumes: WHIMS-MRI study. *Neurology* 2014 Feb 4;82(5): 435–442.

Richter Y, Herzog Y, Cohen T, et al. The effect of phosphatidylserine-containing omega-3 fatty acids on memory abilities in subjects with subjective memory complaints: a pilot study. *Clin Interv Aging* 2010 Nov 2;5:313–316.

Richter Y, Herzog Y, Lifshitz Y, et al. The effect of soybean-derived phosphatidylserine on cognitive performance in elderly with subjective memory complaints: a pilot study. *Clin Interv Aging* 2013;8:557–563.

Shaw K, Turner J, & Del Mar C. Tryptophan and 5-hydroxy-tryptophan for depression." In Shaw, Kelly A. Cochrane Database of Systematic Reviews 2002 (Online); (1):CD003198.

Sigala S, Imperato A, Rizzonelli P, et al. L-alpha-glycerylphosphorylcholine antagonizes scopolamine-induced amnesia and enhances hippocampal cholinergic transmission in the rat. *Eur J Pharmacol.* 1992 Feb 18;211(3):351–358.

Vakhapova V, Cohen T, Richter Y, et al. Phosphatidylserine containing omega-3 fatty acids may improve memory abilities in nondemented elderly individuals with memory complaints: results from an open-label extension study. *Dement Geriatr Cogn Disord.* 2014 Feb 20;38(1-2):39–45.

Vakhapova V, Cohen T, Richter Y, et al. Phosphatidylserine containing omega-3 fatty acids may improve memory abilities in non-demented elderly with memory complaints: a double-blind placebo-controlled trial. *Dement Geriatr Cogn Disord* 2010; 29(5):467–474.

Xing SH, Zhu CX, Zhang R, et al. Huperzine A in the treatment of Alzheimer's disease and vascular dementia: a meta-analysis. *Evid Based Complement Alternat Med* 2014; 363985. Epub 2014 Feb 3.

Zhang Y, Leung DYM, Richers BN, et al. Vitamin D inhibits monocyte/macrophage proinflammatory cytokine production by targeting mapk phosphatase-1. *Journal of Immunology,* 2012 March 1.

Zhang Z, Wang X, Chen Q, et al. Clinical efficacy and safety of huperzine alpha in treatment of mild to moderate Alzheimer's disease, a placebo-controlled, double-blind, randomized trial. *Zhonghua Yi Xue Za Zhi.* 2002 Jul 25;82(14): 941–944.

Chapter Five

American Physiological Society. Aerobic exercise may improve non-alcoholic fatty liver disease. *ScienceDaily* 13 April 2011.

Ancoli-Israel S. Sleep and aging: prevalence of disturbed sleep and treatment considerations in older adults. *J Clin Psychiatry* 2005;66 Suppl 9:24–30; quiz 42–43.

Anderson D, Seib C, & Rasmuss L. Can physical activity prevent physical and cognitive decline in postmenopausal women? A systematic review of the literature. *Maturitas* 2014 June 13.

Avidan AY. Epidemiology, assessment, and treatment of insomnia in the elderly: epidemiology of insomnia in the elderly. Medscape Multispecialty: http://www.medscape.org/view article/516282_2.

Crooks VC, Lubben J, Pettiti DB, et al. Social network, cognitive function, and dementia incidence among elderly women. *Am J Public Health* 2008 Jul;98(7):1221–1227.

Freed B & McCarthy WJ. Low aerobic fitness and obesity are associated with lower standardized test scores in children. *J Pediatr* 2010 May;156(5):711–718, 718.e1.

Gibbons TE, Pence BD, Petr G, et al. Voluntary wheel running, but not a diet containing (-)-epigallocatechin-3-gallate and beta-alanine, improves learning, memory and hippocampal neurogenesis in aged mice. *Behav Brain Res* 2014 Jul 5;272C:131–140.

Halpern J, Cohen M, & Kennedy G. Yoga for improving sleep quality and quality of life for older adults. *Altern Ther Health Med* 2014 May-Jun;20(3):37–46.

Henning CH, Zarnekow N, Hedtrich J, et al. Identification of direct and indirect social network effects in the pathophysiology of insulin resistance in obese human subjects. *PLoS One* 2014 Apr 7;9(4):e93860.

Holt-Lunstad J, Smith TB, & Layton JB. Social relationships and mortality risk: a meta-analytic review. *PLoS Med* 2010 July 27; 7(7).

Iwasa H, Yoshida Y, & Kai I. Leisure activities and cognitive function in elderly community-dwelling individuals in Japan: a 5-year prospective cohort study. *J Psychosom Res* 2012 Feb;72(2):159–164.

Jin Y, Hendrie HC, Liang C, et al. Late life leisure activities and risk of cognitive decline. *J Gerontol A Biol Sci Med Sci* 2013 Feb;68(2):205–213.

Katzman R, Terry R, DeTeresa R, et al. Clinical, pathological, and neurochemical changes in dementia: a subgroup with preserved mental status and numerous neocortical plaques. *Annals of Neurology* 1988; 23(2):138–144.

Laurin D, Verreault R, Lindsay J, et al. Physical activity and risk of cognitive impairment and dementia in elderly persons. *Arch Neurol* 2001 Mar;58(3):498–504.

Leininger S & Skeel R. Cortisol and self-report measures of anxiety as predictors of neuropsychological performance. *Arch Clin Neuropsychol* 2012; 27(3):318–328.

Mahncke HW, Bronstone A, & Merzenich MM. Brain plasticity and functional losses in the aged: scientific bases for a novel intervention. *Prog Brain Res* 2006;157:81–109.

Miller MA, Wright H, Ji C, et al. Cross-sectional study of sleep quantity and quality and amnestic and non-amnestic cognitive function in an ageing population: the English Longitudinal Study of Ageing (elsa). *PLoS One.* 2014 Jun 26; 9(6):e100991.

Nakamura K & Meguro K. Relation between dementia and circadian rhythm disturbance. *Nihon Rinsho* 2014 Mar;72(3): 579–584.

Pace-Schott EF & Spencer RM. Age-related changes in the cognitive function of sleep. *Prog Brain Res* 2011;191:75–89.

Sanchez-Espinosa MP, Atienza M, & Cantero JL. Sleep deficits in mild cognitive impairment are related to increased levels of plasma amyloid-beta and cortical thinning. *Neuroimage* 2014 Sep;98:395–404.

Scarmeas N, Cosentino S, Portet F, et al. Leisure activity and cognitive decline in incident Alzheimer disease. *Arch Neurol* 2007 Dec;64(12):1749–1754.

Wang HX, Jin Y, Hendrie HC, et al. Late life leisure activities and risk of cognitive decline. *J Gerontol A Biol Sci Med Sci* 2013 Feb;68(2):205–213.

Wendell CR, Gunstad J, & Waldstein SR. Cardiorespiratory fitness and accelerated cognitive decline with aging. *J Gerontol A Biol Sci Med Sci.* 2014 Apr;69(4):455–462.

Wilson RS, Krueger KR, Arnold SE, et al. Loneliness and risk of Alzheimer disease. *Arch Gen Psychiatry* 2007 Feb;64(2):234–240.

Yaffe K, Weston A, Graff-Radford NR, et al. Association of plasma beta-amyloid level and cognitive reserve with subsequent cognitive decline. *JAMA* 2011 Jan 19;305(3):261–266.

Index

About the Author

Earl Mindell RPh, MH, PhD, is an internationally recognized expert on nutrition, drugs, vitamins, minerals, and herbal remedies. Dr. Mindell is often called the Father of the Nutritional Revolution. In 1971, Dr. Mindell co-founded a chain of vitamin stores. He is the author of fifty-six health-oriented books that have been translated into thirty-four languages worldwide, including the all-time bestselling nutritional book *The New Vitamin Bible,* which has sold over 11 million copies. Some of his other books include *Herb Bible, Prescription Alternatives, Supplement Bible,* and *Anti-Aging Bible.*

Dr. Mindell is a registered pharmacist, master herbalist, and holds a Ph.D. in nutrition. He has been awarded the President's Citation for Exemplary Service from Bastyr University for his contributions to the health and well-being of humanity. He was inducted into the California Pharmacists Association Hall of Fame 2007 and was awarded the President's Award from the National Nutritional Food Association. He is also on the Board of Directors of the California College of Natural Medicine and serves on the Dean's Professional Advisory Group, School of Pharmacy, Chapman University 2014.

Dr. Mindell served on the International Board of Nutrition for Nestle International for six years. He spoke with Get Motivated from 1999 to 2009 with such luminaries as Colin Powell, Rudy Giuliani, Zig Zigler, President George Bush, Margaret Thatcher, President Gerald Ford, Elizabeth and Bob Dole, William Shatner, and Christopher Reeves. He has appeared on *The Oprah Winfrey Show, Live with Regis and Cathy Lee, Good Morning America,* CNN, and *The Late Show with David Letterman* and has been on more than 300 radio and TV shows worldwide.

OTHER TITLES BY DR. EARL MINDELL

Dr. Earl Mindell's Natural Remedies for 150 Ailments

Earl Mindell, R.Ph., Ph.D.

This updated and expanded edition shows you how to stop turning to potentially harmful medications to ease your ailments—and to turn instead to safe, natural, and effective remedies to relieve troublesome health conditions.

320 PAGES • 6 x 9 • ISBN: 978-1-59120-118-2

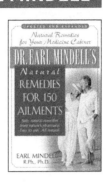

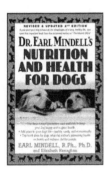

Dr. Earl Mindell's Nutrition and Health for Dogs 2nd Edition

Earl Mindell, R.Ph., Ph.D., and Elizabeth Renaghan

This updated edition discusses easy, flexible, and affordable ways to keep your dog healthy, and elaborates on the different nutritional requirements and specific health issues of different breeds.

256 PAGES • 6 X 9 • ISBN: 978-1-59120-203-5

GOJI: The Asian Health Secret

Earl Mindell, R.Ph., M.H., Ph.D.

Goji is the most nutritionally dense food on the planet and goji extract makes it convenient and easy to get the benefits of this amazing food. Learn how goji extract can unleash your body's potential for a full and healthy life.

64 PAGES • 5-1/4 X 8-1/4 • ISBN: 978-1-59120-315-5

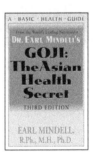

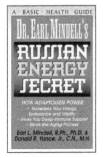

Dr. Earl Mindell's Russian Energy Secret

Earl Mindell, R.Ph., Ph.D. & Donald R. Yance, Jr., C.N., M.H.

In this guide, you'll learn how adaptogen power increases your energy, endurance, and vitality; gives you deep immune support; slows the aging process; enhances health and well-being; and increases your ability to cope with stress.

48 PAGES • 5-1/4 x 8-1/4 • ISBN: 978-159120-000-8

Easing the Pain of Arthritis Naturally
Earl Mindell, R.Ph., Ph.D.

In this book, Dr. Mindell presents safe, easy-to-use strategies to help achieve optimum health and relief. This book features arthritis-busting dietary recommendations to cleanse the body of toxins and introduces superfoods for alleviating symptoms. Anyone who suffers from arthritis will find this book invaluable.

176 PAGES • 6 X 9 • ISBN: 978-1-59120-109-0

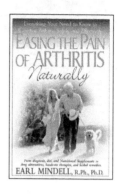

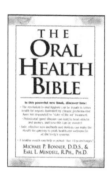

The Oral Health Bible
Michael P. Bonner, D.D.S.
& Earl L. Mindell, R.Ph., Ph.D.

This informative book contains an action plan for taking charge of our oral health and educates us and our physicians and dentists on how many debilitating health problems are intimately linked to oral health and hygiene.

144 PAGES • 6 X 9 • ISBN: 978-1-59120-050-5

Greens Are Good for You!
Earl Mindell, R.Ph., Ph.D.
& Tony O'Donnell

This book tells how greens can protect against heart disease; cancer; diabetes; macular degeneration; poor night vision; senile dementia; liver disease; fatigue; and blood, sleep, urinary, and colorectal disorders.

48 PAGES • 5-1/4 X 8-1/4 • ISBN: 978-1-59120-036-9

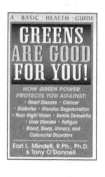

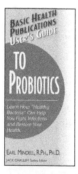

User's Guide to Probiotics
Earl Mindell, R.Ph., Ph.D.

"Good" bacteria populate our digestive tract, help us maintain normal digestion, and protect us against stomach flus, candida overgrowth, and many types of infections. In this concise book, Dr. Mindell explains the many health benefits of probiotics—and how to use them to enhance health.

96 PAGES • 3-3/4 X 8-1/2 • ISBN: 978-1-59120-114-4

VISIT WWW.BASICHEALTHPUB.COM